# Starting and Maintaining a Successful Dermatology Practice

*Editor*

BRETT COLDIRON

# DERMATOLOGIC CLINICS

www.derm.theclinics.com

*Consulting Editor*
BRUCE H. THIERS

October 2023 • Volume 41 • Number 4

**ELSEVIER**

1600 John F. Kennedy Boulevard ● Suite 1800 ● Philadelphia, Pennsylvania, 19103-2899

http://www.theclinics.com

**DERMATOLOGIC CLINICS Volume 41, Number 4**
**October 2023 ISSN 0733-8635, ISBN-13: 978-0-443-18318-8**

Editor: Stacy Eastman
Developmental Editor: Nitesh Barthwal

*Dermatologic Clinics* (ISSN 0733-8635) is published quarterly by Elsevier Inc., 360 Park Avenue South, New York, NY 10010-1710. Months of publication are January, April, July, and October. Business and editorial offices: 1600 John F. Kennedy Blvd., Suite 1800, Philadelphia, PA 19103-2899. Customer service office: 11830 Westline Drive, St. Louis, MO 63146. Periodicals postage paid at New York, NY, and additional mailing offices. Subscription prices are USD 438.00 per year for US individuals, USD 899.00 per year for US institutions, USD 478.00 per year for Canadian individuals, USD 1,097.00 per year for Canadian institutions, USD 536.00 per year for international individuals, USD 1,097.00 per year for international institutions, USD 100.00 per year for US students/residents, USD 100.00 per year for Canadian students/residents, and USD 240 per year for international students/residents. International air speed delivery is included in all *Clinics* subscription prices. All prices are subject to change without notice. **POSTMASTER:** Send address changes to *Dermatologic Clinics*, Elsevier Health Sciences Division, Subscription Customer Service, 3251 Riverport Lane, Maryland Heights, MO 63043. **Customer Service: 1-800-654-2452 (U.S. and Canada); 314-447-8871 (outside U.S. and Canada). Fax: 314-447-8029. E-mail: journalscustomerservice-usa@elsevier.com (for print support); journalsonlinesupport-usa@elsevier.com (for online support).**

*Reprints.* For copies of 100 or more, of articles in this publication, please contact the Commercial Reprints Department, Elsevier Inc., 360 Park Avenue South, New York, New York 10010-1710. Tel.: 212-633-3874; Fax: 212-633-3820; Email: reprints@elsevier.com.

The *Dermatologic Clinics* is covered in *MEDLINE/PubMed (Index Medicus), Current Contents/Clinical Medicine, Excerpta Medica, Chemical Abstracts,* and *ISI/BIOMED.*

# Contributors

## CONSULTING EDITOR

**BRUCE H. THIERS, MD**
Professor and Chairman Emeritus, Department
of Dermatology and Dermatologic Surgery,
Medical University of South Carolina,
Charleston, South Carolina, USA

## EDITOR

**BRETT COLDIRON, MD, FACP, FAAD**
Clinical Associate Professor, University of
Cincinnati, The Skin Cancer Center, Cincinnati,
Ohio, USA

## AUTHORS

**BRADFORD E. ADATTO, JD**
Partner, ByrdAdatto, Dallas, Texas, USA

**RICHARD G. BENNETT, MD**
Bennett Surgery Center, Santa Monica,
California, USA; Department of Dermatology,
Keck School of Medicine of USC, University of
Southern California, Division of Medicine
(Dermatology), David Geffen School of
Medicine, University of California, Los Angeles,
Los Angeles, California, USA

**ROBERT T. BRODELL, MD**
Tenured Professor and Chair, Department of
Pathology, Professor and Past Founding Chair,
Department of Dermatology, Billy S. Guyton
Distinguished Professor, University of
Mississippi Medical Center, Jackson,
Mississippi, USA

**JOSHUA BURSHTEIN, MD**
National Society for Cutaneous Medicine,
Department of Dermatology, Mount Sinai Icahn
School of Medicine, New York, New York, USA

**MICHAEL S. BYRD, JD**
Partner, ByrdAdatto, Dallas, Texas, USA

**BRETT COLDIRON, MD, FACP, FAAD**
Clinical Associate Professor, University of
Cincinnati, The Skin Cancer Center, Cincinnati,
Ohio, USA

**MARTHA LAURIN COUNCIL, MD, MBA,
FAAD, FACMS**
Former President, St. Louis Metropolitan
Medical Society, Washington University in St.
Louis, St Louis, Missouri, USA

**KRISTINA M. DERRICK, MD**
Clinical Instructor, Department of
Dermatology, SUNY Downstate Health
Sciences University, New York Harbor
Veterans Administration - Brooklyn Campus,
Brooklyn, New York, USA

**ALEXANDRA FLAMM, MD**
Assistant Professor of Dermatology, NYU
Grossman School of Medicine, Department of
Dermatology, Penn State Health, Hershey,
Pennsylvania, USA

**CAROLE C. FOOS, CPA**
Principal, OJM Group, LLC, Cincinnati, Ohio,
USA

**JOSEPH FRANCIS, MD**
Department of Dermatology, University of Florida College of Medicine, Gainesville, Florida, USA

**NICOLE M. GOLBARI, MD**
Clinical Instructor, Department of Dermatology, SUNY Downstate Health Sciences University, New York Harbor Veterans Administration - Brooklyn Campus, Brooklyn, New York, USA

**GEORGE J. HRUZA, MD, MBA, FAAD, FACMS**
Laser & Dermatologic Surgery Center, Chesterfield, Missouri, USA; Adjunct Professor of Dermatology, St. Louis University, St. Louis, Missouri, USA

**PAYVAND KAMRANI, DO**
Department of Dermatology, Penn State Health, Hershey, Pennsylvania, USA

**SAILESH KONDA, MD**
Department of Dermatology, University of Florida College of Medicine, Gainesville, Florida, USA

**BARRY LESHIN, MD**
Chapel Hill, North Carolina, USA

**LANA L. LONG, MD, FAAD**
Assistant Clinical Professor, University of Kentucky, Private Practice, City Dermatology & Laser, Cincinnati, Ohio, USA

**DAVID B. MANDELL, JD, MBA**
Partner, Principal, OJM Group, LLC, Cincinnati, Ohio, USA

**JASON M. O'DELL, MS, CWM**
Principal, OJM Group, LLC, Cincinnati, Ohio, USA

**KISHAN H. PANDYA, MD**
Transitional Year Intern, Summa Health System, Akron, Ohio, USA

**DAVID M. PARISER, MD, FAAD, FACP**
Private Practice, Professor, Department of Dermatology, Eastern Virginia Medical School, Norfolk, Virginia, USA

**SAGAR PATEL, MD**
Department of Dermatology, University of Florida College of Medicine, Gainesville, Florida, USA

**DARRELL RIGEL, MD, MS**
Dermatologist, National Society for Cutaneous Medicine, Department of Dermatology, Mount Sinai Icahn School of Medicine, New York, New York, USA

**DANIEL M. SIEGEL, MD, MS (Management and Policy)**
Clinical Professor, Department of Dermatology, SUNY Downstate Health Sciences University, New York Harbor Veterans Administration - Brooklyn Campus, Brooklyn, New York, USA

**ROBERT SKAGGS, MD, FAAD**
Dermatology, University of Kentucky College of Medicine, Kentucky Skin Cancer Center, Cincinnati, Ohio, USA

**JERRY D. SMITH, MD**
Fellow of the American Academy of Dermatologists (FAAD), Clinical Professor, The University of Texas Southwestern Medical Center, Dallas, Texas, USA; Director, Medical Arts Clinic, Corsicana, Texas, USA; Founder, LCS Free Skin Cancer Screening Clinic, Ajijic, Jalisco, Mexico

**CYNDI YAG-HOWARD, MD, FAAD**
CEO, Yag-Howard Cosmetic Dermatology, Associate Professor, University of South Florida Morsani College of Medicine, Naples, Florida, USA

**DANNY ZAKRIA, MD, MBA**
Dermatology Resident, National Society for Cutaneous Medicine, Department of Dermatology, Mount Sinai Icahn School of Medicine, New York, New York, USA

# Contents

Robert Skaggs and Brett Coldiron

Opening a small private dermatology practice can be a rewarding experience. It may seem like a lot of trouble, but in no other setting will you have so much freedom, control, and directly be able to see the consequences of your efforts. Economically, you must realize that in other settings, all these "chores" you must do in a solo practice are paid for by you out of overhead, which can greatly exceed what it costs if you do it yourself in a small practice. That is, a small private practice can be economically more rewarding and flexible than working for a dermatology group, particularly a multispecialty group. It requires months of preparation, planning, hard work, persistence, and a strong desire to establish a practice that operates on your own terms.

Bradford E. Adatto, and Michael S. Byrd

This chapter will provide guidance on the steps a dermatologist should consider when starting a new practice or adding a new partner. Additionally, this chapter details the tools a physician can use to evaluate the various types of "entities", which are sole proprietorship, general partnership, corporations, and limited liability companies. Furthermore, this chapter examines the four primary areas that tend to determine whether the parties are sufficiently aligned for success. These four areas -The 4 C's are (1) Cost; (2) Compensation; (3) Control and (4) Contingencies.

Kristina M. Derrick, Nicole M. Golbari, and Daniel M. Siegel

Understanding the economics behind any medical practice comes down to one basic concept: Profit = Revenue – Expenses. This article aims to demystify the details that underlie this simple formula and to provide the budding dermatologist the information and the tools needed to determine their own profitability in the "real world."

Barry Leshin

There are a variety of practice models to select from as we establish the framework that optimizes our practice of medicine. Work satisfaction is closely connected to the right fit of the model selected. A model of increasing popularity is the private equity backed dermatology practice management (DPM) company. The objective of this chapter is to describe this model and how it can provide a meaningful pathway.

Private equity's (PE) presence has grown within dermatology over the last decade, creating a new landscape for dermatologists to navigate. Although dermatology PE-backed groups (DPEGs) claim to partner with physicians and improve health care delivery, their actions show that investment returns and profits are prioritized. The history of PE in medicine, the corporate practice of medicine, maturation of the dermatology market, monopolistic practices, overleveraging of nonphysician practitioners, dependence on debt, training under PE, and professional and lifestyle considerations are discussed. Dermatologists should be wary of DPEGs in order to protect the profession and patients.

The retirement process is an individualized endeavor. Both financial and social aspects are important to consider when making plans for retirement. In this article, we discuss details of retirement planning, including the need to save, how much and when to start saving, and types of retirement plans. We also review key considerations for deciding when to retire as well as aspects of retirement outside of financial planning, such as redefining one's purpose and finding meaningful activities to fill the void of work.

Dermatology referral utilization is increasing, with 15% of dermatology-related visits by primary care resulting in a dermatology referral. Given this, both strengthening an expanding a referral is a key component of a successful dermatology practice. In particular, effective communication is essential for efficient patient-oriented coordinated care. Written and/or verbal communication can help build a strong communication network and, in some instances, can be applied toward Merit-based Incentive Payment System (MIPS) reporting and billing for coding families that incorporate the coordination of care. Reaching out directly to referring clinics has also been shown to increase the quantity of referrals. This can include providing clinics with patient handouts on your clinic, education on what information is prioritized within the referral, and educating staff on how to complete their referrals effectively and efficiently. Social media can play an important role in referrals, especially for patients looking for cosmetic care. There are many different platforms, and these can serve as a marketing tool for physicians looking to bring in new patients.

The reality of dermatology practice in the 21st century includes the potential for lawsuits and liability. While medical malpractice may be top-of-mind, there are a host of liability risks beyond malpractice–from employee claims and fiduciary liability for the practice retirement plan to premises liability and HIPAA violations–as well as potential personal liability for rental properties, car accidents (for self and children), outside businesses, personal guarantees and more. This article outlines the leading tools dermatologists can utilize to better shield their assets from potential liability–including exempt assets, co-ownership forms, and legal tools, such as limited liability companies and trusts.

# DERMATOLOGIC CLINICS

---

SERIES OF RELATED INTEREST

*Medical Clinics*
https://www.medical.theclinics.com/
*Immunology and Allergy Clinics*
https://www.immunology.theclinics.com/
*Clinics in Plastic Surgery*
https://www.plasticsurgery.theclinics.com/
*Otolaryngologic Clinics*
https://www.oto.theclinics.com/

# Preface

# Is Private Practice a Possibility for Me?

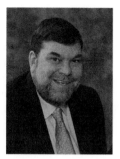

Brett Coldiron, MD, FACP, FAAD
*Editor*

Whether you are coming out of residency or considering your options as you transition from one job to another, the option of private practice (solo or group) may have crossed your mind. This collection of essays should inform and perhaps inspire you to consider private practice.

You may not have any entrepreneurial spirit, and you may just want to clock in and out. This sounds nice, but you will become aware that there is a high price to pay in loss of autonomy and income. If you shoulder the administrative chores, your career rewards may be much greater. I believe private practice is the best way to practice. It allows for the greatest personal freedom, and most importantly, allows you to provide the best possible care for your patients.

In this issue, the basics of starting your own private practice or joining one are covered in detail. The pitfalls to avoid and personal mistakes we all made are shared, and resources to make informed decisions are included. For example, it may seem odd to cover retirement planning in the same space as starting a practice, but this is a crucial topic to consider at the beginning of a career, even if you never plan to retire.

Personally, I started in academic medicine and then transitioned to private practice, which was the best decision I have ever made. It has afforded me great joy and success, allowing me to make my own decisions, achieve financial independence, and still be an advocate for the specialty.

There is a lot of business preparation you need to succeed at in private practice, and much of this, and resources for more, are in this issue. One of my exasperated former trainees who went and set up his own private practice flattered me by confiding, "you make all this seem so easy!" It seemed easy because of personal experience and getting the right people to work for me, which I think is the hardest part.

Some tips I would add are, when you are still a resident or even medical student, to work with some private practitioners, and if they are agreeable, emulate them, copy their office manuals, and photograph their setups, supplies, and sources. All of the authors in this issue would be happy to give you advice. Even easier is to take over or join a private practice and step into their groove. As you gain control, you can make changes you want without having to re-create things from scratch.

Established private groups also may have more remunerative contracts with private insurers. Negotiating with insurers can be difficult, and better contracts are valuable. Be aware that if your focus is skin cancer, however, your biggest (and unfortunately often the best) insurer will be Medicare, with rates that are set by the federal government for each area, and that most private insurers, including Medicare advantage plans, set their reimbursement as a percentage of Medicare. The other most difficult issue, at least for me, is human

Dermatol Clin 41 (2023) xi–xii
https://doi.org/10.1016/j.det.2023.07.003
0733-8635/23/© 2023 Published by Elsevier Inc.

resources, that is, hiring the right employees and maintaining them.

The tremendous debt most residents carry is a great detriment to the specialty, forcing residents to make some difficult, if not downright unsavory choices. One point that is mentioned herein needs to be emphasized. If you take a position without long-term intentions, make sure you can leave when you intend to. You must give careful consideration of noncompete clauses, which will remain effective for the foreseeable future, and avoid anchoring your personal life.

The pros and cons of working for private equity are discussed in detail in this issue, and the only caveat I will add is they can be valuable in a crowded market area, especially if they have better insurance contracts. I would note that most of them do not have better contracts, and this is an issue to explore in some detail.

I hope you enjoy this issue and do not feel obligated to read cover to cover, as it is designed for perusing. I hope our efforts inspire and enable young and seasoned Dermatologists to consider private practice.

Sincerely,

Brett Coldiron, MD, FACP, FAAD
University of Cincinnati
The Skin Cancer Center
3024 Burnet Avenue
Cincinnati, OH 45219, USA

*E-mail address:*
bcoldiron@gmail.com

# Starting a Solo Practice

Robert Skaggs, MD[a],*, Brett Coldiron, MD[b]

## KEYWORDS

• Career • Young dermatologist • Solo practice • Private practice • Purpose-driven

## KEY POINTS

- Starting a solo practice takes courage, determination and perseverance.
- About 57% of dermatologists consider themselves to have ownership in their practice, and even fewer are solo owners of their practice.
- Despite the challenges of modern medicine, starting your own dermatology practice is doable and is a very rewarding and enriching style of practice.

## INTRODUCTION

Every young dermatologist in the final year of residency or fellowship looks at the next step in their career. Our lives to this point have been purpose-driven; we had to get into college, get into medical school, excel so that we could have our choice of residency position, and then learn about the skin so that we could take great care of our patients and future patients. Where and in what setting you take care of those patients is a difficult decision for most dermatologists exiting their training.

Dermatologists have significantly more employment options than many of our other physician colleagues. To name a few, dermatologists can join an academic center, a large group, a small group, private-equity or physician owned, concierge/cash-based, cosmetic, military, or start their own practice. According to the 2020 AAD Member Profile, two-thirds of AAD members were in either a solo or group practice.[1] About 57% of dermatologists consider themselves owners of the practice they work in, whether as owners, shareholders, or partners.[2] This group of dermatologist-owned, private-practice dermatologists is getting smaller every year.[1,2]

I remember asking my fellowship director for employment advice, long past when most of the dermatology fellows and residents in my year had signed their respective contracts, if I could have a private practice like the one he created. Politely and directly, he said: 'You have to want it.' At that moment, it clicked for me, and I knew I wanted 'it'. I decided to start a solo practice near my hometown.

Starting your own practice is an exciting career move that can be fulfilling. You learn business skills, make a positive meaningful impact on your community, and do it on your own terms. This is enticing, but it requires arguably more planning, hard work, and dedication than the other options discussed above.

## WHERE DO YOU START?

The American Medical Association has a terrific series of podcasts that cover how to start a medical practice. They are highly recommended as a good starting place.[3]

### Location/Market Analysis

As soon as you decide to start your own clinic, you must get the ball rolling quickly. One of the most important decisions is determining what community your practice will be in. Most often, dermatologists choose communities close to their family/friends or in places with amenities they desire.

[a] Dermatology, University of Kentucky College of Medicine, Kentucky Skin Cancer Center, 1818 Wallace Court, #301, Bowling Green, KY 42103, USA; [b] University of Cincinnati, Skin Cancer Center, 3024 Burnett Avenue, Cincinnati, OH 45219, USA
* Corresponding author. Dermatology, University of Kentucky College of Medicine, Kentucky Skin Cancer Center, 1818 Wallace Court, #301, Bowling Green, KY 42103.
E-mail address: Robertskaggs5@gmail.com

Dermatol Clin 41 (2023) 557–564
https://doi.org/10.1016/j.det.2023.04.001
0733-8635/23/© 2023 Elsevier Inc. All rights reserved.

However, an important consideration is how much your future community needs dermatology care or what the market demand is for a dermatologist. Most dermatologists flock to coastal and metropolitan cities, but the biggest market demand is often in smaller communities.

You should consider how many patients are in the area you are considering compared with the number of dermatologists available. Not only that, but you should also investigate what types of insurance/payors are present in the community. Important factors are the percentage of Medicaid, HMO, PPO, and Medicare beneficiaries in the area, median income in the area, the education level, and the economic trajectory of the community. If you want to open a cosmetic, boutique practice, it would not be prudent to open your practice in an impoverished town with a declining population. Providing dermatologic care to any community is worthwhile, but it is important to make sure your vision of your dermatology practice fits with the community you are considering.

### Name/Company Description

Choosing a name is an important step in determining the trajectory, branding, and reputation of your practice. If you know you want to be a solo practitioner, perhaps 'Your Name Dermatology' is a good option. However, if you want to hire other dermatologists, it may be harder to bring them onboard if they are working for 'Your Name'. Consider the services you will offer, the location of your practice, and how you want to brand your practice.

1. Choose something simple and memorable
2. Include services offered
3. Target audience
4. Check availability
5. Feedback, feedback, feedback

If your practice has a focus like pediatrics, cosmetics, or surgery, make sure to allude to it with your name, but avoid narrowing the scope of your services. Make sure that the name you want is available in your state by accessing the secretary of state's office. Equally important is checking to see if the domain name and social media handles you want are available. Lastly, ask people you trust what they think of your choice of a practice name. Often, they will provide a perspective different from yours, which can be helpful.

I chose to name my practice 'Kentucky Skin Cancer Center' because I saw it as a fantastic, direct representation of the mission of my practice. This was similar to the name of the practice from my fellowship, and I saw how patients identified with the name of the practice. The feedback I received from my advisors was that 'Cancer' was a forbidding choice to include. However, I trusted my instinct and have found that patients with skin cancer seek out my practice, which was the intended purpose.

Developing a mission statement is another important step in establishing your practice's identity. This is a short statement or paragraph that states the goals of the practice and the way it will accomplish them. This is an integral foundation for your staff and your branding, a sort of message from the heart about your practice vision.

### Develop a Business Plan

Once you get to this point, you need to determine how to finance the start of your practice, how you will generate revenue to cover your expenses, and ultimately be able to pay yourself at some point along the way. There are many public resources available on the American Academy of Dermatology Web site and at local universities. I reached out to a small business development department at a local university. Most public schools have a version of this available to the public for free. They can help you develop projections on your income, expenses, start-up costs, profit and loss statements, and balance sheets.

All these types of documents will be critical to get funding from a lender so that they can be assured your business model will be successful. Of course, if you have another source of capital to finance the start of your practice, you may not need a lender. In general, it is recommended to plan to have 6 months of operating expenses available for your practice. Depending on your payor mix and credentialing, it may take 6 months before you will be paid for your work as you start seeing patients.

Business development plans will be different for everyone and every practice. Some will envision a no-frills, low overhead practice, and others will desire posh, boutique practices. No matter what you choose, it is always wise to be conservative with your projections to give room for error and financial shortcomings. It is common to have delays and setbacks from the conception of your practice to opening the doors for your first patients. No matter what your plan is, have a direction and go with it.

### Find a Place of Business

The physical location of your practice is critical to the success of your practice. You want to make sure the quality of construction, the quality of surrounding tenants, accessibility, location demographics, and visibility meet your standards.

I learned some hard lessons when finding a place of business for my practice. For the most part, altruism and collegiality are common qualities in medicine. Those qualities are often lacking in the business world, where 'it's just business' is a common phrase. Often other parties are solely looking for their best interests, and that means you must do your homework and be prepared with contingency plans.

It is a good idea to find a real estate broker or someone you can trust to help guide you through the purchase or lease of a space to start your practice. There are many variables here most do not learn in college or medical school like buildout allowances, commencement dates, initiation dates, triple-net versus gross leases, common property, and renewal options. Real estate sellers and landlords often have partners, make sure to know who the decision-makers are and be thorough in your specific requests for your practice.

I signed my lease and found out later that a main competitor in town was best friends with one of the owners of my leased space. My landlord reduced my parking, didn't allow my signage to say my practice name, and generally tried to hinder my success.

You will also need to have a general contractor and an architect or designer if your space needs improvement before seeing your first patients. It is important to work closely with the architect to make sure your space will fit your needs. Most architects have not built out a dermatology space and won't know as much as you do about your practice needs. Get multiple contractors to bid on your construction project and sign an agreement that protects you. My general contractor backed out of the project 1 week before construction starting. If you don't have an agreement with them, you have no recourse. Having multiple contractors bid on the project helps you have a way to manage construction costs and protect your timeline for opening your doors.

## What Services Will You Offer

All board-certified dermatologists have received quality training and can perform many dermatologic services. However, in the beginning, it is important to have a wider focus, which you can narrow as you build your practice. General dermatology is foundational in most practices. From this base, you can expand your services as needed.

A few months after my practice opened, I discovered I had received minimal revenue due to a credentialing error and found myself in a budget crisis. We had purchased equipment and supplies to process permanent section biopsies in house, along with lots of other equipment for general and surgical dermatology. To make payroll for my employees, I had to sell the permanent section equipment back to our supplier for 60% of what I had paid for it 6 months prior. I had never used the equipment. It was necessary to do this, but it would not have been if I had waited to purchase the equipment when I was ready to use it. More importantly, you need to pursue your credentialing at least as aggressively as monitoring your construction build out. Local or state medical societies often provide a credentialing service for members, and there are other sources.[4,5]

The services you offer in year one may be different from what you can offer in the following years once you have solidified your practice. Many dermatologists have training and interest in laser treatments, but lasers are typically expensive and take a while to show a return on investment. Lasers or other expensive equipment can be useful in your practice, but make sure your patient population can support them before committing your start-up capital. There are laser rental services in many areas, and you can have them dropped off and picked up for a day or a half day a few times a month. These can be expensive, and you may find it cheaper to partner up with another physician or two and share a device.

## Credentialing

This is crucial to your financial success if you take insurance payments for your services. At a minimum, you need a physical address, a National Practitioner Identification (NPI) number, a Drug Enforcement Agency (DEA) number, a state medical license number, malpractice insurance, and a phone number to provide to the insurance company so that they can verify that your business is legitimate. Many insurance companies require more than this, but this is a starting point. These are all time-consuming and must proceed in a certain order. You should allow at least 6 months to obtain these. In addition, these items can be expensive, with a medical license costing several hundred dollars and the DEA recently raising its 3 year charge to $888.[6]

The National Institute of Health defines credentialing as 'a formal process that utilizes an established series of guidelines to ensure that patients receive the highest level of care from healthcare professionals who have undergone the most stringent scrutiny regarding their ability to practice medicine'.[3] This is what credentialing is from the insurance companies' perspective. However, for a practice owner, credentialing is often a barrier between patients and the dermatologist.

Insurance companies can change plan types from year to year and require you to become credentialed with each new plan type. All too often, these plans have narrow networks, which requires you to keep a watchful eye on the plans offered to your patients by the various insurance companies.

Credentialing, once you have all your paperwork in order, always takes several weeks, and it commonly takes several months to get approved as an in-network provider. You can do this yourself if you have the time to dedicate to it. As mentioned above, local and state medical societies or even third-party vendors may provide credentialing services for you. There is a charge for any of these, and be aware that you may have to get recredentialed regularly. Buyer beware, this is a critical part of your new practice survival, and you will need to monitor the progress being made regularly.

My personal experience with a third-party contractor nearly doomed my practice from the beginning. Most insurance companies require mountains of paperwork to verify to the clients/patients in their network that you are, in fact, a legitimate business and dermatologist. Unfortunately, our credentialing third-party contractor put an incorrect address on one of the many, many documents sent back and forth. This caused 80% of the revenue we generated in our first 6 months to be 'frozen' until our mailing address could be reverified. During this process, a 90 day hold was placed on all payments to our practice. After the 90 day hold, we had to call their customer support lines and request 2 to 3 payments at a time. I had an employee work 40 hours per week for 4 weeks on this project.

You should ensure you have someone with great attention to detail handling your credentialing to avoid a similar nightmare scenario.

### Negotiate with Insurance

Negotiating an insurance contract is a complex, time-consuming, daunting, but necessary process for every practice. For fee-for-service insurance based medical practices, you cannot adjust prices to meet demand or cover expenses like other businesses do in basically every other industry. Your revenue, excepting noninsured cosmetic procedures, is constrained by the insurance contracts in your area. It is difficult to get favorable terms and reimbursement rates. Often, insurance companies will not negotiate with start-up medical practices and a basic contract is all that is offered. However, it never hurts to ask, and with many insurance companies, you may find an opportunity to negotiate. You may find that there are insurances that pay so poorly that you do not want to participate

with. Be aware that many commercial insurances now administer Medicaid under attractive names but still pay poorly.

First, you can confidentially ask a trusted colleague in the area what the market rates are in your area. There are also commercial insurance databases, such as MGMA.[7]

This will also give you an idea of what is reasonable to expect from insurance companies and if you have any room to bargain with them. You should learn what the benchmarks are in your area. Most insurance companies pay as a 'percentage of Medicare' rates. Knowing what your Medicare reimbursement rate is in your location is the first item to become familiar with. Medicare rates can be found at the Medicare Web site.[8,9]

Do not be disheartened if you cannot get the same rates as the local multispecialty practices or large groups. Typically, they have much higher overhead, and what insurers pay them and what they receive from the group may be less than what you ultimately receive. You should also realize that more than half of your payer base will probably be Medicare. Whereas Medicare usually pays less than commercial insurance, it pays punctually every 2 weeks and does not have as many obstacles to care, such as prior authorizations.

Do your homework on your practice and write down what your strengths are. If the insurance company would not negotiate with your start-up practice, be ready after year one to show them how your practice benefits their clients. Items to consider are your service area, how many patients are in your practice, demonstrated patient satisfaction, relative expertise, note your competitors, affiliations, the health benefits you provide to their clients, and the services you provide.

Before starting negotiations, see if you have any connections to the decision-makers at the insurance company. Ideally, you should establish rapport with the insurance company before negotiations. You should find out if there is something you can offer that will benefit them. Even better, if there are large employers in your area, introduce yourself to the one or two people in the human relations department who are responsible for health insurance purchasing. They have tremendous clout with commercial insurance companies, and if you can convince them of your value to their employees, you have a valuable ally. Employers care most about employees missing work but also about the cost if they are self-insured. Attending local health fairs is a good way to establish relationships and identify who the big local players are.

Next, find out who you will be negotiating with, do some research on them, and set up a time to discuss your requests. Prepare a detailed proposal and explain why you deserve what you are asking for. You should be prepared to answer questions about your proposal as needed.

These discussions are often stressful, and it is important to always remain professional. At times, there may be long delays in communication, which can be unnerving. Being persistent and positive is a good approach to maintaining constructive dialogue. Ultimately, you must make good decisions to maintain the health of your practice. A compromise is usually necessary to find an agreement.

In times when an agreement is not easily found, walking away is sometimes the best choice. As the practice owner, it is sometimes necessary to walk away from a contract with poor rates or conditions. Make sure to keep your global business strategy in mind. You will be surprised at how good you get at this as you go along.

Insurance negotiation requires research, careful planning, and persistent communication. Keeping a clear focus on your goals can pay dividends for your practice if you are successful. Every effort you make can be fruitful, improve your financial position, and help you take care of your patients more easily.

### Hire a Team

When you are weeks to months away from opening your doors, you need to hire employees to join your practice. Before you do, it is a good idea to know the number and types of employees you need to start. Market research will show you what the compensation and benefit packages are for these positions in your area. Once you have this information, you can model what your labor costs will be and what you can afford. Please keep in mind that if your practice expands, your number of employees will grow, and thus the cost of the benefits and hourly compensation/salary will grow significantly. As a small business owner, you must be prepared to step into any roles you want to hire employees to fill.

You may also want to consider offering incentives such as flexible schedules to attract and retain top talent. Remember that working in a dermatology office is often a desirable position with unexpected fringe benefits like happy patients/clients, no working nights, weekends, or holidays, complimentary cosmetic services, and skin care services and products. This can work in your favor and allow you to gain quality employees who may be able to earn more elsewhere.

Research any minimal educational requirements for your office employees through your state medical board and state government Web sites. For example, there may be requirements if you will be drawing blood in your office. A few states require histotechnicians to have a minimum amount of post-high school education.

Familiarize yourself with the labor laws in your area before interviewing and hiring employees. There are questions you cannot ask a potential hire in an interview. Specially, it is illegal to ask about age, genetic information, birthplace, country of origin, citizenship, disability, gender, sex or sexual orientation, marital status, family situation, pregnancy, race, color, ethnicity, or religion.

When you are interviewing employees, make it clear what your expectations are and how you will evaluate their performance. You write this out first, and even better, have it all in print in an employee office manual. The American Academy of Dermatology has an office policy and procedure manual that provides a nice template.

The group of individuals you hire will likely have more contact with your patients than you will, so make sure they will represent your practice the way that you want them to represent you. It is important for your initial success to have a friendly, competent team.

### Purchasing Equipment

Every practice has basic equipment and supply needs to get started. Many companies and distributors will offer start-up allotments and deals. You should get price quotes on all of your items from multiple vendors. They will likely help you greatly because there is a long list of items you will need to get started, and medical supply companies are used to and eager to help start-up practices.

Price shopping and planning with multiple vendors can be a good way to decrease your overhead and minimize the cost of your start-up equipment. Most vendors are vying for your business and want to establish a long-lasting partnership that benefits parties. You may find doing business with one main vendor or splitting your purchases with multiple vendors is best for your practice. Whatever you find, it is important to establish a relationship with these vendors, so it is easy to communicate when supplies are low or there are back orders on items you need. For example, there are certain vendors who can obtain local anesthetic whereas others cannot. You may also, however, find you can meet most of your needs through online sources.

Starting equipment like patient chairs, electrosurgical equipment, and surgical tools come in different quality and cost categories. Depending on your vision for your practice, you may choose to go with new equipment, inexpensive equipment, or refurbished equipment. Wholesale companies exist that buy equipment and supplies from practices that close or decide to upgrade. These items are often in high demand because they are less expensive than new items. You can get examination tables reupholstered on site for a reasonable price.

Dermatology conferences are great places to meet many different vendors and see what their equipment offerings are. Here you can look, touch, and use the equipment to see the quality and cost. Equipment purchases are an easy way to ramp up start-up costs, so be conservative and purchase only what you know you will need. Always ask for the "convention special". This is usually an additional 10% off the quoted price.

Business items you will need to purchase are computers, phone systems, tablets if you have an electronic medical record (EMR) system, printers, shredders, fax machines, Internet supplies, and a refrigerator or other appliances for the staff break room. Many retail stores have holiday sales, so consider timing your purchases around these sale periods.

Set a budget for your equipment purchases and stick to it.

### Develop a Marketing Strategy

If you are starting a practice from scratch, marketing your practice is crucial. If you have no starting patient base, you must find a way to let patients know what you do, where you are, and that you are available to help them. Marketing is a competitive and changing area, so it is important to stay up to date and relevant.

You must decide what your "brand is," develop a logo, and promote it. You can do this yourself or tap into the local graphic design class at the community college. Have some fun, but once decided, stick to it.

First, consider your patient population and how they interact with advertisements. You need to know if your patients are young versus old, rural versus urban, and what their exposures are. When considering advertisements, you should keep in mind your advertisement goal. You may want the patient to visit your Web site or call your office for an appointment. Make sure your advertisement will accomplish your goal. The first advertisement we used displayed our practice name and 'coming soon'. It was less than ideal because there was no phone number, no Web site address, or any actionable way for the viewer to learn more about us. A Web site should come first. Recall that you can schedule patients several months in advance of the actual opening. Ideally, you should be able to collect most information online before scheduling but in an older population, you will be doing most of this on the phone. Consider what kind of on hold message or music you want, if any. Phone on hold is a possible time to tell patients of the additional services you offer or tout your training.

Social/digital media are modern ways of advertising and can be used to target certain demographics. You can create content to target certain populations or, more simply, you can create basic content to direct traffic to your practice Web site or phone number. Elderly patients are sometimes not familiar with social media platforms. You will likely need to use alternative media to reach them. Whereas yellow page entries are largely obsolete, a one-line listing in the yellow pages and the white pages is inexpensive and essential. Beware the useless solicitations for special Internet or "national business" yellow page listings that seem to be bills. You may need a consultant for digital ads that will pop up on smart phones and interactive radio stations. Do set up Internet feedback sites and ask happy patients to rate you.

Newspapers can be a useful way to reach older patients. You can create more informative content for newspaper ads because the viewer has more time to look at the ad and there is potentially more space to add content. Be sure to find out what the exposure of said newspaper is. If you are in a large city, the newspaper may reach many people who are 'out of your area'. If you are in a small city, the newspaper may be effective.

Billboards are a great way to raise awareness that your practice exists. Be sure to show your logo or practice name, what you offer, and how to find you or reach your office. Radio ads are another way to target drivers, particularly older ones who listen to talk radio.

Television is a robust way to advertise, but it can be expensive. With streaming television, active demographic targeting is possible but technically difficult. Content creation for television advertisements is harder to create than most of the other forms of advertisements mentioned above.

Perhaps the best form of advertisement is through physician and patient referrals. Patients trust their primary care physicians and providers to make good decisions about their specialists. Their opinion matters a great deal to your potential patients. If you can gain the trust of a primary care physician, you may get a steady stream of patients into your office.

Whatever your advertising plan is, stick to it, because this is the only way your practice will grow in the beginning.

## Hit the Ground Running/Train Your Team

Now that you have everything in place to start your practice, you will need to tie up the loose ends to start taking care of patients. The American Academy of Dermatology has many resources to help with onboarding employees and training strategies.[5] You will want to establish written protocols for the different duties and processes in your office before interviewing.

A decision must be made on whether you will document with paper charts or with an EMR. Paper is much easier and less expensive, but it will result in lower Medicare payments. EMRs are great for claims audits because they force you to record all needed information, and an electronic chart note can be quickly sent for record requests. EMRs, however, are expensive, costing an average of $32,000 per provider per year.[10] and may have additional storage or user fees. Some EMRs may have integrated billing and quality improvement reporting. Be aware that the EMR company technically owns your data, and it may almost be impossible to separate from them in the future. Many EMR companies will do on-site training for your team. Recall, however, that as a small practice, it will fall to you to become the expert in its use and be able to train new employees.

One of the most important things you will need to establish is an Employee Handbook. The AAD has a great policy and procedure book with a useful template.[11] This will be a governing document for employee benefits, expectations, how to take care of patients, and how to request time off. Check with a local employment attorney or other business owners for their handbooks. You may also want to consult with a human resource officer to help with your Employee Handbook. We used the human resource officer with our office health insurance broker to help us establish our Employee Handbook.

You will also want to walk your employees through the patient experience at your office and let them know what your expectations are of them. Training your team on the small things in your office, like how to answer the phone, how to greet patients, and how to care for the patients in your office, can help build your office culture and brand your practice.

## SUMMARY

Opening a small private dermatology practice can be a rewarding experience. It may seem like a lot of trouble, but in no other setting will you have so much freedom, control, and directly be able to see the consequences of your efforts. Economically, you must realize that in other settings, all these "chores" that you must do in a solo practice are paid for by you out of overhead, which can greatly exceed what it costs if you do it yourself in a small practice. That is, a small private practice can be economically more rewarding and flexible than working for a dermatology group, particularly a multispecialty group. It requires months of preparation, planning, hard work, persistence, and a strong desire to establish a practice that operates on your own terms. The path to becoming a successful practice will require overcoming challenges and perseverance. Ultimately, establishing a practice of your own and making an impact on the community I live in has proven to be rewarding.

## CLINICS CARE POINTS

- About 57% of dermatologists consider themselves owners of the practice they work in, whether as owners, shareholders, or partners.
- The number of dermatologist-owned, private-practice dermatology clinics is getting smaller every year.
- Starting a solo practice is a challenging, multifaceted experience that will take a team of trusted individuals to accomplish your goal.
- There are many resources at local colleges and at in professional medical and dermatology organizations that help you along the way.

## DISCLOSURE

The authors have nothing to disclose.

## REFERENCES

1. Available at: https://assets.ctfassets.net/1ny4yoiyrqia/1msGYRRlqVuy8VNhEl1kME/94294769ff3c7a30a397e50bb04d8a15/Practice_Models_White_Paper_V231.pdf. Accessed April 15, 2023.
2. Available at: https://www.aad.org/dw/monthly/2019/june/private-equity-at-a-glance. Accessed April 15, 2023.
3. Available at: https://www.ama-assn.org/practice-management/private-practices/expert-tips-help-doctors-navigate-private-practice-challenges. Accessed April 15, 2023.
4. Available at: https://www.ncbi.nlm.nih.gov/books/NBK519504/#:~:text=Credentialing%20is%20a%20formal%20process,their%20ability%20to%20practice%20medicine. Accessed April 15, 2023.

5. Available at: https://www.aad.org/member/practice. Accessed April 15, 2023.

6. Available at: https://www.federalregister.gov/documents/2020/03/16/2020-05159/registration-and-reregistration-fees-for-controlled-substance-and-list-i-chemical-registrants. Accessed April 15, 2023.

7. Available at: https://mgma.com/?utm_source=digital&utm_medium=search&utm_campaign=bra-gen-feb-2023-mgmabrand&gclid=Cj0KCQjw2v-gBhC1ARIsAOQdKY0FRst-jYT41QchXtjFDBYUgIBGGS9ZIU686b_5f–BdK_YYqJt6UgaAjLgEALw_wcB. Accessed April 15, 2023.

8. Available at: https://www.cms.gov/medicare/physician-fee-schedule/search/overview. Accessed April 15, 2023.

9. Available at: https://www.cms.gov/medicare/medicare-fee-for-service-payment/pfslookup. Accessed April 15, 2023.

10. Available at: https://www.commonwealthfund.org/publications/newsletter-article/cost-biggest-barrie-electronic-medical-records-implementation. Accessed April 15, 2023.

11. Available at: https://shop.aad.org/products/dermatology-office-policy-procedure-manual. Accessed April 15, 2023.

# Basic Legal Considerations in Starting and Maintaining a Dermatology Practice

Bradford E. Adatto, JD[1],*, Michael S. Byrd, JD[1],*

## KEYWORDS

- Dermatology practice • Forming a corporation • Manager-managed LLC • General partnership
- Sole proprietorship • Limited liability partnership

## KEY POINTS

- Various factors must be considered when opening a dermatology practice, whether you have already begun, are currently in the process, or just dreaming of starting one.
- Forming a professional entity presents unique challenges, requiring specialized knowledge to navigate the process successfully and efficiently.
- There are benefits and differences between a limited liability company (LLC) and a corporation.
- It is important to be aware of the pros and cons before adding a business partner(s).
- Seek legal counsel to help form and run a successful dermatology practice.

## INTRODUCTION

The thrill of starting a dermatology practice can be intoxicating. Starting up a business allows the physician to have their own practice by themselves or with other key individuals to launch the brand and ideas. However, the choice a physician must make on forming the right entity and partnering with the right physicians can sometimes be petrifying. Some dermatologists may have already launched their practice but now are weighing if they considered all of the options. Others are ready to start another ancillary business such as a medical spa and need to better understand what was missed the first time. This article provides guidance on the steps a dermatologist should consider when starting a new practice or adding a new partner.

## DISCUSSION
### Formation of New Practice

In most situations and states, a dermatology practice requires formation of a professional entity.

Professional entities are entities formed for the purpose of providing a professional service, such as medical services rendered by a physician or group of physicians. This article does not attempt to discuss every state possibility but provide a general introduction into each entity type. In addition, forming a professional entity can bring about unique challenges and therefore requires special knowledge to navigate both successfully and efficiently. Each state has rules and regulations on the types of professional entities that may be formed and who can own or co-own with the particular professional entity. There are several professional entities recognized by the states, which include professional associations, professional medical corporations, service corporations, and limited liability partnerships. For example, in New York, the options for professional entities include professional corporations (also called domestic professional service corporations) and professional limited liability companies ("LLC"), whereas in Texas the types of professional entities that may be formed include professional associations and

ByrdAdatto, PLLC, Dallas, TX 75206, USA
[1] Present address: 8150 N Central Expy, Suite 930, Dallas, TX 75206, USA.
* Corresponding authors.
E-mail addresses: badatto@byrdadatto.com (B.E.A.); mbyrd@byrdadatto.com (M.S.B.)

Dermatol Clin 41 (2023) 565–571
https://doi.org/10.1016/j.det.2023.07.001

derm.theclinics.com

professional LLCs. Finally, in California a partnership or a professional corporation may be used. California uniquely does not recognize professional LLC as an appropriate entity to provide medical services.

Once the applicable entity is chosen, one typically must form the entity with the secretary of state and obtain an employer identification number from the Internal Revenue Service. This article focuses on the most common business types of "entities," which are sole proprietorship, general partnership, corporations, and limited liability companies.

### Corporations

The corporation is one of the oldest business entities offered in all states. Although it can be a rigid entity choice with plenty of hoops to jump through and maintain, the corporation has been consistently used for decades and comes with a well-developed body of law. The entity can be used for any size of business ranging from one owner to the Wall Street public corporation with thousands of owners. Many states allow professionals to form professional corporations, service corporations, or professional associations, which are generally treated as a specific type of a corporation. As such, a professional corporation formed for the purpose of providing professional service will still follow the same principles of a corporation but will have additional restrictions on ownership and control (Fig. 1).

**Formation** Depending on the state, the filing of a Certificate of Formation, Articles of Incorporation, or Articles of Formation with the Secretary of State is the first step in forming a corporation. The owners of a corporation, called shareholders, are issued stock and elect directors to serve on the board of directors. Typically, it is the board of directors that approves business decisions and elects the officers of the corporation, who run the day-to-day operations. The officers serve at the pleasure of the board of directors, and the board of directors serve at the pleasure of the shareholders. Under many state laws, at least one President and one Secretary, who can be the same person, must be elected.

The primary organizational documents that should be in place and will need to be analyzed for a corporation are the bylaws (adopted by the board of directors) and shareholders agreement (adopted by the shareholders). The bylaws will typically address the basic operational, management, and wind-up procedures, whereas the shareholder agreement will contain the transfer restrictions on shares and voting powers given to the

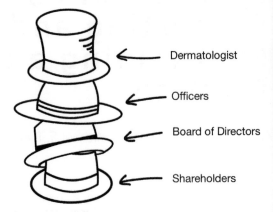

**Fig. 1.** Corporations.

shareholders. The shareholders agreement is also where the shareholders can determine how much power will be given to the directors by restricting their rights to approve certain business actions without shareholder's prior approval. Examples of such restrictions would be matters relating to the sale of the corporation or sale of substantially all of the assets; this typically is proportional to the number of shareholders: the more shareholders there are, the more independence and power the directors will have and vice versa.

**Liability** Forming a corporation allows for a shareholder to shield themselves from being personally liable for the corporation in most instances. Stated another way, if the corporation was to be sued, the shareholders' investments in the corporation could be at risk, but their personal assets outside the business would likely be protected. Incorporation will not protect you from malpractice claims but will protect your personal assets if someone falls in the waiting room.

In addition, the directors have a reduced liability for the decisions they make in regard to running the corporation. It is well established that directors are fiduciaries of the corporation, but they owe the duties of care and loyalty to the corporation and not the shareholders themselves. Their decisions must be those that they deem to be in the best interest of the corporation, but the business judgment rule provides a secondary level of protection. It states that as long as directors and officers of a corporation can justify their actions as being in the honest pursuit of business, they have not breached their duty to the corporation.

**Tax Election** Another choice in developing a corporation is tax election. Once the corporation is formed, a corporation may be taxed at the entity level (ie, a "C" corporation ("C Corp")) or on a pass-through basis at the shareholder level (ie, a subchapter "S" corporation). Accordingly, the "C" corporation designation is merely a federal tax classification where the company will be taxed based on its corporate income. Most companies that are publicly traded on the stock exchanges are C Corps; however, publicly traded companies constitute less than 1% of all US businesses.

A subchapter "S" corporation ("S Corp") is federal tax classification where the corporation itself is not taxed at the entity level, but income, losses, deductions, and credits are passed through and taxed at the shareholder level based on each shareholder's own tax bracket. S Corps, however, have several limitations, which may affect their feasibility when selecting this structure for a new business. Shareholders may only be natural persons, certain types of trusts, estates, and certain exempt organizations (such as a 501(c)(3) nonprofit), but cannot be partnerships, corporations, or nonresident aliens. Further, an S Corp may have no more than 100 shareholders, all of which must be US citizens or residents, and it may have only one class of stock with profits and losses allocated in proportion to each shareholder's percentage interest of ownership. It is strongly suggested that a CPA or tax advisor be consulted in making tax decisions.

### Limited Liability Companies

Limited liability companies ("LLCs") are comparatively one of the newer entity options and are also one of the most popular. An LLC will limit personal liability in a similar fashion as an S Corp. The LLC is a flexible entity, whose attributes are a blend between a corporation and a partnership, but can be customized toward being more like one than the other as desired by its owners. Because of this range of different organizational styles that can occur, it is important to treat each LLC on a case-by-case basis and not make any assumptions as to how it is organized. Much similar to professional corporations, many states allow professionals to practice in professional LLCs, or in some states a regular LLC (**Fig. 2**).

**Formation and Management Structure** The LLC is formed by filing a Certificate of Formation or Certificate of Incorporation depending on the state. The owners of an LLC are called members, and one of the first choices to be made is which management style to adopt: to either run the entity via the members or appoint managers to do so on behalf of the members. The options are member-managed or manager-managed.

The first option is called a member-managed LLC. In this management style, members hold the ownership interest in the entity and retain

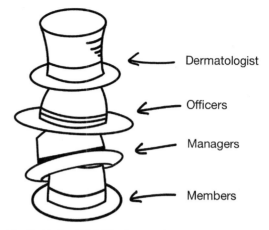

Fig. 2. Limited Liability Companies.

complete control over the management of the entity. The members can either split the management evenly among themselves or designate one or more to be the managing member(s). It is important to understand that in a member-managed LLC, the members' names may be listed with the secretary of state as is the case in Texas, and these members can bind the company to any obligations.

The second option is called a manager-managed LLC. Under this option, the members appoint at least one manager. It is worth noting that the managers do not need to be members of the company. Much like the directors of a corporation, the managers can be given as much or little power to act unilaterally as the members' desire. Generally speaking, the idea is that the managers handle the operations of the business without needing ownership approval but would need authorization to make certain major decisions such as selling the company. These parameters are described in the governing document for the LLC, often known as an operating agreement. In some states, the operating agreement is referred to as a company agreement or regulations.

**Liability Shield** LLCs provide a liability shield for their members. Generally, state law will note that a member or manager is not liable for debt, obligation, or liability of an LLC, even if under a judgment or court order. However, the company agreement can override this term and provide a different liability structure, so it is important to pay close attention to any liability provisions.

**Tax Election** Another area of flexibility found with the LLC is its ability to choose a tax structure either as a disregarded entity, partnership, C Corp, or S Corp; this is often referred to as the "check-the-box" option on tax elections. Approximately 92% of private businesses in the US are structured from a tax perspective as pass-through entities such as partnerships, subchapter "S" Corp, and proprietorships. This means that income from your practice will be taxed as if directly received by you. It is strongly suggested that a CPA or tax advisor be consulted in making tax decisions.

As the option for the structure of the dermatology practice is narrowed based on the differences in formation, liability, and tax options, the physician should consider the structure of how the owners plan to govern their practice.

### General Partnership

A general partnership ("*GP*") is similar to a sole proprietorship ("SP"), except there are 2 or more people as owners rather than one. Importantly, each partner has *unlimited* personal liability for the entire liability of the GP. Parties can agree in writing under a partnership agreement to limit each partner's liability. However, this does not prevent employees, patients, or other third parties from filing actions or claims against one or all of the partners for all of the liability. GPs do not file any formation documents with the secretary of state to start a GP. A GP in many states can be formed by oral agreement. However, written partnership agreements are always recommended to capture the relationship of the partners. The partnership agreement should detail (1) rights to the share of the profits; (2) expressed intent to create a partnership; (3) shared control of business; (4) sharing of losses and liabilities; (5) indemnification between the parties; and (6) joint contribution of money and/or assets to the business. Because of the unlimited liability, it is not recommended that any physicians form a GP as a choice of "entity." Many states do allow a professional limited liability partnership ("*LLP*") to be formed. This LLP has many of the same rules of a GP, but it does limit the liability of each partner by law versus indemnification between the partners. The LLP, where allowed, typically does require a state filing to receive the benefits of liability protections for the owners.

### Sole Proprietorship

The most simple and easy-to-maintain "entity" choice is the sole proprietorship. To be clear, this is not an "entity" but an idea. This election is the default classification for a business. The business typically is a single-owner business that does not take any steps to incorporate. The business can register to use a trade name or "doing business as" name, but the business does not exist separate from the person. For example, all income from the business is taxed as if it was the owner's personal income. With only one owner in an SP, the entity does not require large amounts of maintenance or documentation to run, but there is an important trade off—there is no liability shield between the business and the owner. This lack of a liability shield exposes the owner of an SP to *unlimited* personal liability for the business's actions and debts; this can expose you to devastating litigation. In addition, when an owner wants to sell their "business" there is no stock or shares associated with the business. The assets of the business are owned by the individual owner, and therefore, a stock sale could never occur. Consequently, an asset sale is the only structure that can be used to sell an SP business. This sale can cause many issues in the valuation of the business and ability to divide an SP. For these reasons, an SP rarely makes sense as the vehicle to use to start a dermatology practice.

### Adding Partners

In the lifecycle of owning a dermatology practice, it may make business sense at some point to bring in partners. The structure of an ownership arrangement must be rooted in the underlying purpose for adding a new owner. For example, if the purpose in adding a partner is for the new partner to ultimately purchase the entire practice, the design of the arrangement should align with this purpose. Alternatively, the structure may be different when the purpose of adding the physician is for that partner to have some "skin in the game" in the building of the practice. Being in alignment from an expectations perspective going into the partner relationship is imperative. Four primary areas tend to determine whether the parties are sufficiently aligned for success. These 4 areas—the 4Cs—are (1) cost, (2) compensation, (3) control, and (4) contingencies.

### Cost

On the one hand, cost is as simple as it sounds—how much is it going to cost for a dermatologist to become an owner. However, the parties must discuss and understand the details of the price required of a buying dermatologist to become a partner of the practice and what the buying dermatologist will receive in return. The parties must evaluate the actual ownership that is being acquired and the assets and income streams being acquired. For example, a $100,000 sale of 50% of a practice with a high overhead in an "eat what you kill" compensation model with no assets may be overpriced. Yet, a $400,000 price for 50% of a practice with $400,000 a year in profits will pay off in only 2 years.

Similarly, the owner of the practice must contemplate if the ancillary entities will be included in the sale of the practice or a future option-to-buy will be created. For example, if the owner has a separate cosmetic skin business or medical spa, consideration must be given as to whether this will be offered for ownership. This decision again must be grounded in the underlying strategy behind bringing on a new owner in the first place.

It consequently becomes imperative that the owner have a realistic understanding of the value of the practice. The approach and process used to value a practice ranges anywhere from a back of a napkin valuation to hiring one or more certified business appraisers. The valuation of a practice will be based on the fair market value ("FMV") of the practice. To put it simply, FMV is what a willing buyer is willing to buy the practice for and what a willing seller is willing to sell the practice for in an arms-length transaction. Business appraisers will use one of the following 3 approaches, listed as follows, in determining the valuation of a practice. In general, one of the first 2 approaches are used in the valuation of a dermatology practice. The third approach, market approach, is not typically used because there does not tend to be available transactions for sales of practices for an appraiser to rely on as a comparison.

**Cost Approach** With the cost approach, the appraiser will compute the valuation of a practice based on the practice's net asset value (ie, value of assets less liabilities). This approach is commonly used where the value of the practice is devoid of practice good will (ie, goodwill associated with the name and reputation of a practice), and the practice may or may not have professional goodwill (ie, goodwill associated with the name and reputation of the dermatologist). This approach, because most practices do not have a ton of assets, tends to yield a low valuation. The valuation with the cost approach is essentially derived from the balance sheet of the practice.

**Income Approach** The income approach accounts for the revenues, expenses, net income, and profit of the practice, and the appraiser determines a multiple for the valuation. In general, a positive cash flow and a record of net profit generated independent of professional goodwill will increase the multiple and the value of a practice. The valuation of the practice value will also take into consideration the predictability of replicating the positive cash flow in the future. This approach tends to yield a higher valuation but can be a challenge because dermatologists often have a high degree of professional goodwill. An appraiser will

be reluctant to use this approach if the appraiser concludes that the source of the revenues ties mostly to the reputation of the dermatologist. Breaking it down further, the appraiser becomes reluctant if the appraiser concludes that patients would not stay with the practice if the physician owner left the practice.

**Market Approach** The valuation in this approach is based on comparable sales, that is, sale price of other similar medical practices. In industries such as real estate, comparable sales information can be easily derived from publicly traded data. Because medical practices are not publicly traded, data related to comparable sales are difficult to find, and thus this approach is typically not used for valuing a medical practice.

*Compensation*

Compensation, in context to the 4C analysis of areas to discuss for partnership, speaks to compensation among owners of a practice and not compensation under an employment scenario. The partners of the practice must discuss and agree on how to divide the revenue and overhead costs (expenses) of the practice. The 3 basic compensation models seen in dermatology practices are (1) eat what you kill model ("EWYK"), (2) enterprise model, and (3) communist model.

**Eat What You Kill Model** The concept of the EWYK model is that each partner will receive the collections they generate less allocated overhead of the practice. Revenue generated from other sources (assuming these revenue sources are part of the practice revenue and not their own entity) such as a midlevel practitioner, a medical spa, and an ambulatory surgery center must also be allocated. The formula used to share and distribute overhead varies with each practice. Common formulas range from a simple equal allocation of expenses, or the split may be computed using a more complicated formula with multiple methods of dividing various categories of overhead, for example, method A and method B.

Method A: overhead can be divided into (1) direct expenses and (2) shared expenses. Each partner will be responsible for their direct expenses, such as malpractice insurance, salaries of dedicated staff or nurses, and schedulers or practice coordinators specific to the partner. The shared expenses will be split among the partners based on their respective use of the practice's resources, such as common staff, medical supplies, consumables, and other medical inventories. Allocating overhead based on use is generally referred to as "production-based use." So, if a partner produces 60% of the revenue of the practice, then

60% of the production-based overhead will be allocated to that particular partner.

Method B: under this method, overhead can be divided into (1) fixed overhead and (2) variable overhead. Fixed overhead such as rent will be divided evenly among the partners. Variable overhead may be split among partners either (1) based on the partner's production-based use or (2) evenly. In general, production-based sharing of variable overhead would be beneficial to a new dermatologist joining a practice or a senior dermatologist slowing down his/her practice in preparation for retirement.

The EWYK model will generally work best for a single specialty practice rather than a multispecialty practice. In a multispecialty practice with a dermatologist and a plastic surgeon, EWYK can work, but the owners must be particularly attuned to the overhead requirements of each specialty and develop a fair allocation system. Even within a single-specialty practice such as dermatology, one must take into consideration if some partners will primarily perform purely aesthetic cases or some will perform commercial payer cases. Insurance-based cases will generally have a much higher overhead, as these cases require a larger staff to assist with licensure, billing, and collections. Further, commercial payers take anywhere between 60 to 90 days to compensate the dermatologist for the cases.

**Enterprise Model** In this model, each of the partners will make a guaranteed salary and the profits of the practice will either be distributed equally to each partner or shared based on a productivity formula. The guaranteed salary can be allocated equally to each partner or varied based on productivity differences of the dermatologists or on the seniority of the physicians. Generally, compensation is set in this model to account for differences in productivity, and profits are then split according to ownership. This strategy allows the partners who work hardest to be rewarded, yet build value in the form of profits for the ownership in the practice.

Because the compensation in the enterprise model includes productivity as a factor, it works well in most practice environments. The enterprise model will be an ideal compensation model for practices that want to motivate the partners to work together to grow the profits as a team. It is also an ideal choice for practices whose business plan is to grow the brand name of the practice and the practice goodwill. Another advantage of the enterprise model is that business appraisers value practices with an enterprise compensation model higher than practices with an EWYK model.

**Communist Model** The communist model operates as any other traditional nonservice business. Here the partners share the revenues, expenses, and profits equally irrespective of each partner's productivity. As one can imagine, this model is easily susceptible to partner disputes. Typically, practices who deploy the communist model tend to chip away at the model over time by carving out exceptions to compensate for special types of production among the partners. For this model to work, the partners typically must have a deep, trusting relationship. Consequently, this model is commonly seen in husband and wife dermatology practices.

### Control

Decision-making creates another important area of risk in the ownership relationship. The practice must establish who will have the authority to decide and execute (1) day-to-day business decisions and (2) major business decisions for the practice. For example, consider a scenario where one physician practice hires a younger dermatologist to buy-into the practice and ultimately take ownership of the practice. There are numerous ways to structure control over a practice's decision-making issues. Authority may be given to the senior dermatologist to make day-to-day decisions for a certain predetermined period of time. The authority to make and execute the major decisions remains with the senior dermatologist for that predetermined time period, but there may be certain decisions that require both to agree. The practice agreement can be structured to reflect that after the predetermined transition period, the roles are reversed.

Further the practice must also define what will be qualified as day-to-day decisions and major business decisions. This again varies with each practice based on the partner's expectations and vision for the growth of the practice. For example, practice A could define the decision to enter and execute a lease agreement for a $200,000 laser as a day-to-day decision. On the contrary, practice B could state any expenditure more than $5,000 for any purpose is a major decision and therefore must obtain a majority of unanimous approval. Regardless, the owners must communicate and clearly delineate in the medical practice agreement the day-to-day decisions, the major decisions, and the processes to execute them.

### Contingencies

Contingencies are the final C of the 4Cs that owners of a practice must discuss and agree on before entering into a practice agreement. Parties must discuss and decide the terms and conditions that will govern a situation if an unexpected event were to occur. The unexpected events, that is,

"What-Ifs," to name a few are as follows: (1) death of a co-owner; (2) disability of a co-owner; (3) decision of a co-owner to leave the practice; (4) bankruptcy; or (5) divorce of one of the co-owners. Divorce of a co-owner is an important factor to consider, especially in the community property states where each spouse will have equal rights in all earnings; this means that the spouse of the co-owner undergoing divorce may be able to claim a right in the practice. To avoid such scenarios, the practice agreement can proactively include language requiring the spouse of the divorced co-owner to sell back any interest that may be received in the divorce settlement.

It is also imperative for the practice to preplan the valuation method to determine the value of the practice. The valuation of the practice could be based on a (1) predetermined value, (2) predetermined formula, or (3) preagreed on appraisal process. Although the parties are always free to negotiate a valuation of the practice, the pressure created by an unexpected event raises the importance of a preagreed-on fall back approach if the owners cannot agree.

Once the valuation method or purchase price of the practice is established, the next step is to determine the process to buy, sell, and distribute the ownership interest of a co-owner. Most importantly, the practice must decide on if they would be willing to pay the entire buy-out amount in cash at closing or if they would rather establish a cash flow process where a fixed amount with interest will be paid over time. The parties must consider the impact to the practice in such a scenario, as the practice will be losing a revenue stream with the exiting physician and have a financial obligation for the buy-out.

## SUMMARY

When starting a dermatology practice, the physician should pause before they form the entity and first determine how to structure the practice. For those practices that have already launched, refresh the options and confirm that the current model is still important. Finally, there are many more legal hurdles to consider that will be unique to each business and should be discussed with both legal and tax counsel to put oneself in the best position to have the right structure in place to run a successful dermatology practice.

## CLINICS CARE POINTS

Pearls

- It is never too late to plan. A practice will optimize its' business model when the model is tuned to fit the long-term vision of the practice.
- The LLC provides the most flexibility of the choice of entity options.
- Having the 4C conversation among the owners will significantly reduce the risk of a partner breakup.

Pitfalls

- Once a corporation is elected for taxation purposes, it becomes complicated to later switch.
- Stay away from sole proprietorships and general partnerships, as they offer no personal liability protection.

## DISCLOSURE

Bradford E. Adatto and Michael S. Byrd have no relevant financial or nonfinancial relationships to disclose.

# Economics of a Dermatology Practice

Kristina M. Derrick, MD, ScM, Nicole M. Golbari, MD, Daniel M. Siegel, MD, MS*

## KEYWORDS

• Dermatology • Practice economics • Revenue • Expenses • Profitability

## KEY POINTS

- The economics of a dermatology practice requires the understanding of revenue and expenses.
- Once those are unpacked and you determine what you want from a practice, you may use mathematical models to both estimate profitability and model potential earnings.
- Models may also be used to create formulas that compare offers and contracts holistically.

## INTRODUCTION
### Section 1: Envisioning Your Practice

The process of becoming a physician is a relatively clear-cut pathway including undergraduate education, medical school, internship, and at least 3 years of residency training. For physicians nearing completion of their postgraduate training and finally tackling that question of what they want to do with their lives as a "real doctor," many are overwhelmed by choices and their lack of knowledge of the business of medicine. In addition, dermatologists complete their training typically in their early 30s, when they have rising fixed expenses (family, mortgage, student loans) and need to start saving for retirement.

Instead of approaching the job search, interview, comparison, and negotiation process with anxiety or a goal to just finally "make a living," we encourage dermatologists to first reflect on how they envision their ideal practice. Whether the dermatologist uses their vision informally to help in their job search or formalizes it into a business plan for seeking capital to start their own practice, some items are important to consider (**Box 1**).

One of the benefits of the field of dermatology is the tremendous variety in scope, patient age, and types of practice available. Current dermatology residents and recent graduates have universally excelled in academic coursework, published numerous peer-reviewed articles, often participated in running clinical trials or basic science research, and have performed education and community outreach. Many applicants state their desire to stay in academic medicine as a "triple threat" providing patient care, performing research, and teaching. It is fine to accept that goals change and to take a hard look at what your (and your family's) vision of the next 30 years are to help guide you to the best fit for a job. Potential employers will appreciate a physician who has a clear vision for their career and practice type, and a good employer-physician job fit may reduce physician burnout and employer turnover.

After at least 12 years of incredibly hard work after high school, you may just be thinking some version of "Show me the money" (*Jerry Maguire*). Keep in mind that even the worst of jobs in the specialty will put you in the top few percent of wage earners. However, if your goal is to be in the top 0.01%, you are in the wrong profession. Whatever you do, you must understand a simple premise. If you were selling dresses and lost $1 per dress sold and sold a million dresses, you would lose $1,000,000. "Losing the dollar" could be due to not understanding expenses, taxes, employer benefits, or the basic structure of health care payments. In this article, we hope to introduce you to some of these concepts to prepare you to enter

Department of Dermatology, SUNY Downstate Health Sciences University, Brooklyn, NY, USA
* Corresponding author. Department of Dermatology, SUNY Downstate Health Sciences University, 450 Clarkson Avenue, MS 46, Brooklyn, NY 11203.
*E-mail addresses:* cyberderm@dermsurg.org; daniel.siegel@downstate.edu

Dermatol Clin 41 (2023) 573–588
https://doi.org/10.1016/j.det.2023.04.002
0733-8635/23/Published by Elsevier Inc.

**Box 1**
Envisioning your practice checklist exercise

Practice setting

- ☐ Hospital (academic, community)
- ☐ Multispecialty group (physician-owned, private equity–owned)
- ☐ Physician small practice (employed, partner)
- ☐ Solo practice
- ☐ "Privademic": Private practice with variable amount of academic practice (typically precepting a resident clinic 1–4 d per month ± call coverage, either as part-time faculty, adjunct faculty, or voluntary faculty)

Type of work

- ☐ Patient care
- ☐ Research (clinical trials, pharmaceutical trials, chart reviews, case reports)
- ☐ Teaching
- ☐ Consulting (pharmaceutical, cosmeceutical, device, technology, expert soundbites for popular press articles) or employment in one of these industries
- ☐ Administration (within dermatology: medical director of clinic, medical student clerkship director, residency program director, division chief, chair: within system: IRB or research director, Chief Medical Officer, Quality Improvement officer, Clinic or Hospital Director). Although these options are not typically an option for employment directly out of training, they are still important to consider for long term goals

Days/hours per week

- ☐ Full time (typically Monday–Friday, 32–40 scheduled clinic hours, with some call/inpatient consult responsibilities)
- ☐ Part time (3–4 d per week; sometimes scheduled as longer days)
- ☐ Evening or weekend clinics (may be necessary in competitive markets, places without enough clinic space for the number of physicians and other providers)
- ☐ Normal business hours (8 AM–5 PM)
- ☐ Option or requirement for early morning or late evening hours

Location

- ☐ Geographic location (region of country, family and social network, weather, school quality, cost of living, entertainment options)
- ☐ Practice location (density of other dermatology practices or those offering similar services, population size—specialists and cosmetic-heavy practices often need larger or specific populations)
- ☐ Commute (mode of commute, duration, hassle factor, can you work off-peak hours to reduce commute, can you work remotely any of the time [telemedicine, administrative day])
- ☐ Number of locations (how many offices do you need to attend, differences between patients/staff/focus at office)
- ☐ Proximity of hospital(s) if taking call

Types of patients[a]

- ☐ General dermatology in a private practice seeing a variety of adults (skin checks, rashes, acne), children (acne, eczema, warts), surgeries (excisions of cysts, lipomas, and dysplastic nevi), cosmetics (neuromodulators, fillers, lasers, energy-based devices)
- ☐ Proceduralist focus or exclusive (Mohs surgery, excisions, ± cosmetics)
- ☐ Cosmetics only
- ☐ Pediatrics only
- ☐ Other limitations (such as you want to see only adults, no surgeries, no cosmetics)

Nonclinical duties

- ☐ Expectations of practice and yourself for practice building, research/publications, education/mentorship, teaching support staff, running business, consulting
- ☐ Is there protected time and/or salary for these duties, and how does that match with typical time spent on them

[a]We encourage every resident to get as much exposure to all aspects of dermatology and participate in continuing medical education to optimize their chances of feeling comfortable practicing many aspects of dermatology for which they have been trained.

the field better informed of the economics behind our day-to-day practice.

## DEFINITIONS
*Section 2: Understanding Profitability*

Whether comparing offers or trying to build your own practice, it is important to be able to assess your own earning potential. At its most basic, this requires estimates of both your income and your expenses.

A physician's office is unfortunately not as simple a business as a lemonade stand. With the lemonade business, you have low start-up and overhead costs, often not even needing to pay for office space or support staff, and you get paid in full in cash at the time of service. Nevertheless, one basic equation is still crucial to assessing how to succeed in a small lemonade business or a more complicated dermatology practice:

Profit = Revenue − Expenses.

*Revenue*

Therefore, how does a physician actually get paid these days? Mostly through a complex and tedious process of reimbursement through insurance. Yes, there are some practices or services at dermatology offices that are cash only.[1,2] For those, the office staff takes a credit card/cash or enrolls the patient in a third-party financing option. This allows the office to be paid in full at the time of service for what the office has determined is a fair market price for their services. However, for most dermatologists, they will not have the patient base for cash-only care and/or the practice focus that allows for avoiding insurance. Most patients in the United States have health insurance and often pay large premiums; they expect to be able to use their insurance for most of their health care needs.

Nevertheless, insurance payments are not always that simple (**Fig. 1**). As you can see, physician office billing involving health insurance is markedly more complex than an exclusively cash-based business. Waiting months for payments to come through is not unusual. This can be challenging for practices to pay their overhead while awaiting and actively pursuing payment of their insurance claims. Understanding the complexity and length of this process is important for dermatologists who either start their own business or take a contract based on a percentage of collections. If a dermatologist is expecting 45% of collections, but it takes 3 to 6 months to receive the payment from the insurance company, then it will be months before the physician is paid for their work. Physicians joining a group may want to consider having a base salary for this reason.

Physicians starting their own practice should consider working part-time elsewhere and/or obtaining a small business loan and/or line of credit from a bank to help with the first year of start-up costs and delay in revenue. Each of these approaches has its hidden costs, as interest payment scan add up quickly.

In this example, typical of January–March visits when the yearly deductible resets, the insurance pays nothing until the patient has met their deductible. Although the office collected $20 copay on the date of the visit, the office now must collect the remaining $130 from the patient. Some offices may consider keeping a credit card on file with patient's signing authorization to charge based on their insurance explanation of benefits stating what is the patient's responsibility to pay. Other offices may require a certain amount of prepayment, particularly if their office staff determines that the patient has not yet met their deductible for the year. Each insurance contract may vary in whether they allow offices to collect the deductible up front to apply to that visit/procedure.

Let's take a moment to remark on something notable from **Table 1**. The physician set a fee of $400 for their effort in treating the patient, including taking a history and physical examination, reviewing any necessary records, making a diagnosis, discussing treatment options, making a plan, potentially prescribing one or more medications, potentially discussing need for a procedure and its risks/benefits. For this, the physician coded the complexity of their visit as a 99213 (American Medical Association [AMA] Current Procedural Terminology [CPT] codes, reviewed in later discussion) for which, as a reality check, you should be aware in 2023 has a national Medicare average payment rate $85.49. In a direct-pay practice, the physician would state their fee is $400, and the patient would be responsible for all of that. However, when a physician enters an agreement with a health insurance company to be part of their network, they agree to a set of negotiated rates per CPT code. These rates are usually based on a multiplier of Medicare rates, for example, 120% of Medicare if you are in a good market; 50% to 80% if you are not. A physician who sees a patient with this health insurance agrees to accept the rate of $150 for their 99213 visit, and they agree to collect copay at time of visit, and to collect from the patient if the insurance determines it is the patient's responsibility.

Makes you long for the simplicity of the lemonade stand, no? Dr Megan Lewis[3] wrote an article in 2009 explaining "How Doctors Get Paid" and explains why the challenges of payment through health insurance adds many layers of

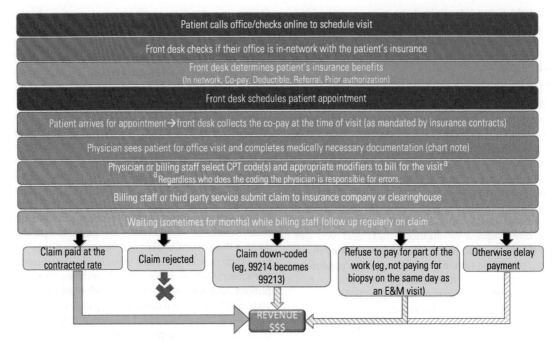

**Fig. 1.** Process for insurance claims.

complexity, increases need for billing and other support staff, and over time prompts physicians to see more patients to cover overhead and retain their income.

One of the most important factors in the success of a dermatologist in being appropriately compensated for their work, regardless of their practice setting, is understanding thoroughly how to code and bill appropriately for their visits and procedures. The AMA created the CPT code set decades ago and continues to create and refine codes to reflect physician work. The American Academy of Dermatology (AAD) has created many resources to understand coding.[4] AAD also has coding and reimbursement Webinars,

Ask a Coder services (coding@aad.org; response within 48 business hours), and Derm Coding Consult columns, such as Dr Alexander Miller's "Cracking the Code" column in *Dermatology World*.[5] The CPT codes for evaluation and management (E&M) coding (99202–99205 for new patients, 99211–99215 for follow-up patients) were revised in 2021 by AMA and further revised in 2023. These codes now prioritize medical decision making to determine the level of the visit, with history and physical examination expected only to the extent medically necessary.

Physicians should take the time to thoroughly understand CPT coding for their office visits (E&M), skin biopsies, and basic procedures along with the proper use of modifiers. Most electronic medical records automatically calculate billing based on documentation in the note, but the physician is responsible for what they charge and should know and agree with the charges submitted under their name rather than accepting the suggested CPT code without review. With regard to cognitive services, EMRs will typically make a selection based on the lowest possible level of coding for a diagnosis. The AMA has an application for smartphones entitled CPT QuickRef (available for both Apple and Android platforms), which has the entire CPT Professional book in the palm of your hand that has a basic free mode and a more extensive paid mode to search for CPT codes.[6]

**Table 1**
**A typical explanation of benefits document may contain this information: current procedural terminology code: 99213 (established patient office or other outpatient visit, 20–29 min)**

| | |
|---|---|
| Physician charge | $400 |
| Insurance contracted rate (allowable charges) | $150 |
| Patient copay (collect at visit) | $20 |
| Deductible remaining | $1000 |
| Patient responsibility | $150 − $20 = $130 |

The Medicare fee schedule is updated yearly to outline payments to physicians for the upcoming year, developed with recommendations from AMA Resource Based Relative Value Scale Update Committee (also known as "the RUC").[7] The value of each CPT code is determined by considering the combination of resources needed to provide the service (Relative Value Units [RVUs]).

1. Physician work: physician time, skill, mental effort (wRVU)
2. Practice expense: staff time, equipment, supplies (PE RVU)
3. Professional liability: cost of associated malpractice coverage (MP RVU)

These factors are then modified based on that site where the service took place ("Non-facility," such as a physician's office, vs "Facility," such as an inpatient hospital or ambulatory surgery center) and the Geographic Practice Cost Index (GPCI), which factors in different costs of overhead, staffing, and supplies in different regions of the country.[8] In addition, Medicare is required to maintain budget neutrality. As spending on health care increases, Medicare reduces physician payments to help achieve this goal, although Congress can override the cut, a common political move almost every year. Every year the conversion factor (CF) is reduced, so the total payment per code typically decreases. For 2022, the CF is $34.61. For 2023, the CF is $33.89.[9]

Simplified, the Centers for Medicare & Medicaid Services (CMS) determines the amount each code will pay using an equation:

Medicare Payment = ((wRVU × work GPCI) + (PE RVU × PE GPCI) + (MP RVU × MP GPCI)) × CF.

As an exercise to better understand this, compare the Medicare payment amount for a 99213 in Manhattan, New York versus Nebraska (Table 2).

RVU values for 99213.

1. Practice expense: 1.26 (nonfacility), 0.55 (facility)
2. Physician work: 1.3
3. Professional liability: 0.10

Therefore, a Medicare payment amount for a 99213 in Manhattan, New York for a nonfacility physician:

1. Practice expense 1.26 (RVU) × 1.203 (GPCI) = 1.52
2. Physician work: 1.3 (RVU) × 1.056 (GPCI) = 1.37
3. Professional liability: 0.10 (RVU) × 2.031 (GPCI) = 0.20

Total
RVU = PE + PW + PL = 1.52 + 1.37 + 0.2 = 3.09.
Payment = Total RVU × CF = 3.09 × $34.61 (for 2022) = $106.99 (slight variation owing to rounding)

In comparison, for a 99214 in Nebraska, for a nonfacility physician, the payment amount is: $85.39.

All of these calculations are done for you and are readily available for any locality though the CMS.gov Physician Fee Schedule Look-Up Tool.[10]

Medicare pays less to facilities for CPT codes because there is less overhead paid by the physician.[11] Hospitals and ambulatory surgery centers often charge a "facility fee" that may make the overall charge to the patient higher than at a private office. Estimated national payments for outpatient procedures, such as skin biopsies and excisions, can be determined based on facility versus nonfacility practice location using the Medicare.gov Procedure Price Lookup tool.[12] For example, for a shave biopsy of the skin (CPT 11102), the average facility cost is $221 (doctor fee, $38; facility fee, $183).

Hospital-employed physicians are often paid with a salary. Hospitals and large groups also have the benefit of size when negotiating for insurance contracts and can often obtain much better contracted rates per CPT code than a solo physician office or small group. This is why Independent Practice Associations/Organizations (IPAs/IPOs) have become more popular, to allow independent physician practices to join together for the purpose of contracting with insurance to obtain better rates.[13] There are also Group Purchasing Organizations, which help practices buy supplies at discounted rates in exchange for fewer choices and more commitment to purchase certain quantities.[14]

IPAs may have membership restrictions and requirements, such as providing hospital call coverage or precepting dermatology residency clinics several times per week. Private insurances often require physicians to have privileges at one or more hospitals in case the patient had an emergency and needed to be admitted. This is rarely needed in dermatology practice and may be negotiable, but physicians who join a medical staff at a

**Table 2**
**For a 99213, the geographic practice cost index modifiers and effect on total Medicare payment are shown**

| Location | Practice Expense | Physician Work | Professional Liability GPCI |
|---|---|---|---|
| Manhattan, New York | 1.203 | 1.056 | 2.031 |
| Nebraska | 0.908 | 1.000 | 0.235 |

hospital will often be required to participate in the call pool.

Private insurances may pay more than Medicare, although in some competitive markets such insurances may pay less. A review by Kaiser Family Foundation found that for all physician services, private insurance paid an average of 143% of Medicare rates (118%–179%).[15] However, most of the studies do not differentiate between facility and nonfacility. Most physicians in the United States are now employed by hospitals or corporate groups (73.9% in 2022).[16]

Every November, in the Physician Fee Schedule final rule, Medicare proposes a cut (eg, 4.5% cut for 2023) in payment for physician services.[17] Any reduction in physician payment by Medicare affects not only Medicare payments but also typically commercial insurance and Medicaid payments, which usually use Medicare CFs and RVU determinations to set their fee schedules in what is essentially an arbitrary decision.

AAD, AMA, and many other physician and hospital groups advocate to Congress yearly to prevent these cuts, usually resulting in a less draconian cut. For 2023, the cut is "only" 2%, but from 2001 to 2021 the Medicare physician payment fell 22% when adjusting for inflation in practice costs.[18] This yearly threat to physician service reimbursement highlights the need for physicians in all practice types to advocate to Congress to avoid these cuts.

Unlike many nonphysician jobs, there is no automatic cost-of-living raise/adjustment for inflation, and year after year the revenue per patient may decrease. These realities force decisions about joining an IPA, selling a practice to a large organization (corporate or hospital), seeing more patients, cutting out the worst insurance payers, increasing patient volume, increasing cash services, reducing support staff, increasing use of midlevels to bill at 85% to 100% rate but with lower salary than a physician, discontinuing hospital consults, and other changes to keep the practice alive. This happens in a solo practice but also in large organizations, where physicians may be expected to add more patients to the day or more clinic sessions in a week.

All medical students and dermatology residents have likely treated many patients who have Medicaid insurance. Medicaid is federally funded health insurance managed by the states primarily for children and indigent people, persons with low income, and persons with disabilities. Many private dermatology practices do not accept Medicaid, based on secret shopper studies of nonacademic dermatologists showing 15% to 20% acceptance of Medicaid, as compared with 92% to 97% acceptance of Medicare and 94% to 98% acceptance of commercial insurance.[19] Although many physicians enter medicine with a passion to help others, and they may desire to help medically underserved patients, as a solo or small practice it may not be financially feasible to take large numbers of Medicaid patients, if any at all. This tool[20] from Kaiser Family Foundation allows you to check the Medicaid to Medicare parity rates. In some states, Medicaid pays the same or higher than Medicare, whereas in others (like New York), Medicaid pays 57% of the Medicare amount for "All services." For example, New York Medicaid rates for physician fees can be viewed online.[21] For comparison, the Medicare Commercial plan (estimated 120% Medicare rates), and Medicaid rates are shown in **Table 3** for a Manhattan physician.

Physician productivity can be measured by how many patients they see, what codes they bill, and what they charge and collect from insurance. However, the amount collected can vary widely by insurance type and payer mix of the practice. Newly hired physicians may be more likely to fill their panels with patients with lower-paying insurance and fewer cash-pay patients. Some practices, especially academic centers, help to equalize this by measuring physician productivity in wRVUs. Employment offers may contain a base salary plus bonus of $50/RVU or similar value. Note the $/RVU offered is usually above the Medicare conversion rate of $34.61 (for 2022). There are many additional pros and cons of RVU-based payment, including not fully capturing all physician clinical and nonclinical work.[22] In dermatology, phototherapy and patch test codes are 2 common procedures that contain no wRVUs, so physicians who are compensated only on wRVUs providing these services may see significant income decreases compared with colleagues whose income is based on collections or total RVUs generated.

How do you increase RVUs (or charges/collections)? See more patients; see patients that require higher medical decision making; or do more procedures. However, always remember the visits and procedures must be justifiable according to medical necessity for insurance to pay and to avoid failing an audit. For example, a patient who wants a benign lesion (seborrheic keratosis, cyst, acrochordon) removed must have documentation of medical necessity (such as pruritus, irritation from clothing, bleeding) and often needs prior authorization. Audits are not uncommon and should not be feared. Instead, you should have pristine and accurate documentation that determines medical

**Table 3**
**Reimbursemnt rates for 99213 in Manhattan in 2022**

| Physician | Location | Facility or Nonfacility | Medicare Payment (2022) | 120% Medicare Payment (Commercial Insurance) | NY Medicaid Payment (2022) |
|-----------|----------|-------------------------|-------------------------|-----------------------------------------------|----------------------------|
| Dr A | Manhattan, New York | Facility | $77.43 | $92.92 | $21.76 |
| Dr B | Manhattan, New York | Nonfacility | $106.99 | $128.39 | $70.76 |

necessity and does not stretch credulity. For example, if every patient is reassured about a benign lesion at every visit to capture an E&M service, that can bring on an audit. If it turns out that every patient on a given day has an angioma on the left shoulder, you could get free lodging in a federal facility.

Another challenge is the multiple procedure payment reduction, where CMS reduces payment for procedures on same day by 50%, with the rationale that there is decremental practice expense or physician work for the additional procedure over the first one. Physicians also must note if they are billing a procedure plus an E&M code, they need

**Box 2**
**Probable expenses**

Practice expenses:

- Physical space (rent/mortgage, electricity, maintenance, association fees)
- Equipment (examination/procedure tables, instruments, autoclave, devices, computers, phones, and so forth)
- Supplies (medication, gauze, alcohol, suture, cleaning supplies, gloves, and so forth)
- Electronic medical records (subscription overall and per provider, IT support) vs paper charts (storage, pay staff for filing and pulling)
- Salaries (office manager, medical assistant, scribe, nurse, other physicians, other providers—PA, NP, aesthetician, virtual assistant)
- Billing (in house vs outsourced—company may take 4%–8% of collections)
- Insurance (property, liability, life, key man insurance)
- Consumables (neuromodulators, fillers, patient-specific or other one-time-use parts for laser and energy-based devices)
- Benefits to employees: retirement plans, health insurance
- Marketing costs (Web pages, mailers, discounts, gifts, search engine optimization, soliciting reviews, social media)
- Reduced price on cash-based services to employees (many practices offer reduced price on cosmetic services to their staff as a benefit and to help them talk about the service to patients)
- Taxation (a good accountant is worth hiring)

Physician expenses:

- Credentialing costs with insurance, IPA fees, hospital staff fees
- Medical license, DEA
- Board certification and maintenance of certification fees
- Continuing Medical Education costs
- Malpractice insurance (occurrence vs claims made policy with tail coverage: more expensive with more years of practice)
- Association dues (American Academy of Dermatology, other specialty societies, local and national medical associations)
- Personal expenses: Auto leases, gym memberships, and so forth
- Taxation (for details, speak to your accountant)

**Box 3**
**Value beyond profits checklist exercise**

Patient load

☐ Number of patients per hour to meet overhead

☐ Time allotted per patient (difference for new vs repeat, difference for procedure or cosmetic)

☐ Ask to see actual physician clinic templates (is there flexibility to change template initially or permanently?)

☐ Hospital call/consults: number and acuity per day, night, weekend, support (residents, midlevels)

Support staff

☐ Number of medical assistants and nurses you will work with

☐ Will your staff be the same, so that you can have consistency ("my Medical Assistant [MA]")?

☐ Who will prepare the tray, get supplies, clean the room between patients?

☐ Who does inbox, prior authorizations, laboratory/biopsy result callbacks, and what is typical volume/time per day per physician?

☐ Is there an MA or a scribe for notes (regardless, always remember that you, the licensed provider, are legally responsible for your coding)?

☐ Do you have input into hiring, reassigning, and firing support staff?

☐ How are challenges, such as staff being sick or short staffing, handled to reduce disruption to physician workflow?

Appetite for marketing

☐ Define your goal with marketing: bringing patients to your practice, building overall practice/department reputation, education outreach, increasing your professional profile, which may have financial and nonfinancial benefits. Many employers require some amount of practice building/marketing

☐ Don't want anything to do with it

☐ Will tolerate occasional video or article by hospital/group marketing team

☐ Want to make some content (blog/Web site articles, social media videos)

Overhead expenses

☐ Do you have to contribute to cosmetic overhead (paying for neuromodulator, filler, and other consumables)?

☐ Are you expected to otherwise contribute to practice overhead?

Income

☐ How will you be paid: salary only, base salary with bonus, percentage of collections, $/RVU, hourly?

☐ For bonus, what are the factors involved (patient volume/income, and at larger groups, may include research, citizenship, and other attributes that help the practice/institution)?

☐ Additional salary for supervising midlevels (physician assistants, nurse practitioners)

☐ Additional salary for practice income not directly related to physician billing codes (eg, patch testing)

☐ Is there an option for partnership? Is there a buy-in? When will the partnership decision be made (typically by 2 y)? What are the expected increased income, other benefits, and duties of a partner?

☐ Is there any plan to sell the practice (is anything under contract), and if there is a sale in the future, how is that negotiated for those who are employees and not partners?

Other financial considerations

☐ Is there a sign-on bonus (may be 5%–20% of salary depending on location)?

☐ Is there any low-interest loan or mortgage assistance?

☐ Are there loan repayment opportunities (Pubic Service Loan Forgiveness–eligible employer, 501(c)3, or government institution; VA loan repayment; organization loan payment—note this is typically taxed just like income vs others are tax-free at least federally)

Continuing Medical Education

☐ Are there any paid days for CME (larger groups may provide 5 d typically)

☐ Are there funds for CME (larger groups may provide $2000–$6000)

☐ Want to become a social media influencer with many followers, potentially paid subscribers and offers of sponsorships

Vacation

☐ Remember that every day you are not in the office, you are not seeing patients and making money. But you/your employer is still paying rent, electricity, supplies, staff payroll, and so forth. The salary an employer gives has factored in vacation and other leave

☐ Are any weeks of vacation guaranteed in contract (private practice standard is 2 wk, some offer 3 wk; academic standard is 4 wk)?

☐ How are vacation and holiday requests handled and prioritized?

Sick leave, including parental leave

☐ Are there paid sick days; do the clinics have to be made up?

☐ Is there flexibility for sick days or days that come up on short notice?

☐ Is there any policy for maternity leave, paternity leave, or caregiver leave?

Payer mix and insurance contracts

☐ What is your practice's mix of private/commercial insurance, Medicare, and Medicaid?

☐ What are your typical insurance rates compared with Medicare (<100% vs >100%)?

☐ Are your physicians in an Independent Practice Association/Organization? What does that mean for insurance contracted rates and are there requirements, such as hospital call coverage?

☐ Are you willing to share some actual physician productivity statements and charges, collections, accounts receivable sheets? (you will most likely need to sign a nondisclosure agreement)

Restrictive covenant/noncompete clause

☐ Is there a noncompete clause?

☐ What distance (urban areas may be measured in blocks or miles; less dense areas may be 5–50 miles)?

☐ What time frame (1 y is typical)?

Other benefits

☐ Health insurance (small practices often cannot afford to offer health insurance to their employees but may offer stipends and employees can find Health Insurance Exchange plans or other plans through various insurance companies)

☐ Dental and vision insurance

☐ Disability insurance and life insurance (physicians should usually have their own plans too)

☐ Discounts to entertainment or item purchases

☐ Retirement plan options and any matching contributions (401(k) or 403(b), 457). What is total amount you can save pretax per year, and does the employer provide a matching contribution and at what percentage (may range from 0% to 10%–20%)?

Professional expenses

☐ Will employer cover the cost of hospital and insurance credentialing, medical license and renewals, DEA license (if applicable), scrubs, lab coat and laundering?

☐ Will employer cover malpractice (occurrence policy or a claims made policy)

☐ Will employer cover malpractice (occurrence policy or a claims-made policy)

☐ Will employer purchase/provide all needed tools for practice (such as a laser or cryostat for Mohs)?

---

to have a separate diagnosis for the procedure versus the E&M code; otherwise, one will not be paid for, unless the necessity is well documented.

Several large groups perform yearly surveys to obtain total compensation and wRVU values for physicians; reports from Medical Group Management Association (MGMA), American Medical Group Association, and Sullivan Cotter may be purchased from those organizations. According to MGMA, the median dermatologist compensation (includes salary, bonus, incentive payments, research stipends, honoraria, and distribution of profits)[23] in 2021 was $498,125.[24] The range within the specialty is tremendous, with the 10th percentile salary $292,150 and the 90th percentile salary $783,554. As you can see, where you fall in this spectrum is influenced by the profits dictated by many of the factors discussed above. However, your final paycheck is not solely based on what you bring in. Understanding and managing your expenses is just as important in calculating your final profit; so, that second part of our equation, (Profit = Revenue – Expenses), should next be explored.

### Expenses

A dermatology practice has many expenses that are necessary to provide care, pay staff, and obtain

**Table 4**
How to calculate your profitability and potential earnings. A few commonly used codes in dermatology practice are shown here to give an idea of the difference between E&M visits and different procedures. For a full list of codes, please see the downloadable file.

| HCPCS Code | Short Description | NonFacility Price | Medicare Multiplier (eg, 1.2×) | Quantity | SOLO | MULTI | TOTAL |
|---|---|---|---|---|---|---|---|
| 99203 | Office o/p new low 30–44 min (E&M) | $112.84 | 1.00 | 0 | x | x | $0.00 |
| 99204 | Office o/p new mod 45–59 min (E&M) | $167.40 | 1.00 | 0 | x | x | $0.00 |
| 99212 | Office o/p est sf 10–19 min (E&M) | $56.93 | 1.00 | 0 | x | x | $0.00 |
| 99213 | Office o/p est low 20–29 min (E&M) | $90.82 | 1.00 | 0 | x | x | $0.00 |
| 99214 | Office o/p est mod 30–39 min (E&M) | $128.43 | 1.00 | 0 | x | x | $0.00 |
| 11102 | Tangntl bx skin single les | $103.36 | 1.00 | 0 | x | x | $0.00 |
| 11103 | Tangntl bx skin ea sep/addl | $51.17 | 1.00 | 0 | x | x | $0.00 |
| 11104 | Punch bx skin single lesion | $128.09 | 1.00 | 0 | x | x | $0.00 |
| 11105 | Punch bx skin ea sep/addl | $60.32 | 1.00 | 0 | x | x | $0.00 |
| 11200 | Removal of skin tags ≤15 | $92.85 | 1.00 | x | 0 | 0 | $0.00 |
| 11301 | Shave skin lesion 0.6–1.0 cm | $124.37 | 1.00 | x | 0 | 0 | $0.00 |
| 11401 | Exc tr-ext b9+marg 0.6–1 cm | $159.27 | 1.00 | x | 0 | 0 | $0.00 |
| 11602 | Exc tr-ext mal + marg 1.1–2 cm | $248.73 | 1.00 | x | 0 | 0 | $0.00 |
| 11641 | Exc f/e/e/n/l mal + mrg 0.6–1 | $241.28 | 1.00 | x | 0 | 0 | $0.00 |
| 11642 | Exc f/e/e/n/l mal + mrg 1.1–2 | $272.11 | 1.00 | x | 0 | 0 | $0.00 |
| 11755 | Biopsy nail unit | $124.37 | 1.00 | x | 0 | 0 | $0.00 |
| 11900 | Inject skin lesions </w 7 | $57.95 | 1.00 | 0 | x | x | $0.00 |
| 12001 | Rpr s/n/ax/gen/trnk 2.5 cm/< | $95.90 | 1.00 | x | 0 | 0 | $0.00 |
| 12011 | Rpr f/e/e/n/l/m 2.5 cm/< | $114.54 | 1.00 | x | 0 | 0 | $0.00 |
| 12032 | Intmd rpr s/a/t/ext 2.6–7.5 | $309.39 | 1.00 | x | 0 | 0 | $0.00 |
| 13101 | Cmplx rpr trunk 2.6–7.5 cm | $404.95 | 1.00 | x | 0 | 0 | $0.00 |
| 13152 | Cmplx rpr e/n/e/l 2.6–7.5 cm | $505.60 | 1.00 | x | 0 | 0 | $0.00 |
| 17000 | Destruct premalg lesion | $68.11 | 1.00 | 0 | x | x | $0.00 |

| Code | Description | Price | | | | | Total |
|---|---|---|---|---|---|---|---|
| 17003 | Destruct premalg les 2–14 | $6.78 | 1.00 | 0 | x | x | $0.00 |
| 17106 | Destruction of skin lesions | $348.36 | 1.00 | 0 | x | x | $0.00 |
| 17110 | Destruct benign lesion 1–14 | $115.56 | 1.00 | 0 | x | x | $0.00 |
| 17261 | Destruction malignant lesion, trunk, arms or legs; 0.6–1.0 cm | $150.46 | 1.00 | x | 0 | 0 | $0.00 |
| 17270 | Destruction malignant lesion, scalp, neck, hands, feet, genitals; ≤0.5 cm | $152.49 | 1.00 | x | 0 | 0 | $0.00 |
| 17281 | Destruction malignant lesion, face, ears, eyelid, nose, lip, mucous membrane; 0.6–1.0 cm | $182.99 | 1.00 | x | 0 | 0 | $0.00 |
| 17311 | Mohs 1 stage h/n/hf/g | $688.59 | 1.00 | x | 0 | 0 | $0.00 |
| 17312 | Mohs addl stage | $418.17 | 1.00 | x | 0 | 0 | $0.00 |
| | DAILY TOTAL | | | | | | $0.00 |
| | 5 d Week | | | | | | $0.00 |
| | 4 d week | | | | | | $0.00 |
| | 4 × 48 wk | | | | | | $0.00 |
| | 5 × 48 wk | | | | | | $0.00 |
| | 4 × 50 wk | | | | | | $0.00 |
| | 5 × 50 wk | | | | | | $0.00 |

*Abbreviations:* o/p, outpatient; E&M, evaluation and management service; mod, moderate; hi, high; est, established; phy, physician (MD or dO); qhp, qualified health care provider (NP or PA); Tangentl, tangential; bx, biopsy; ea, each; sep, separate; addl, additional; incal, incisional; shave, shave removal; exc, excisiontr-ext, trunk, arms or legs; B9, benign; marg, margin; h-f-nk-sp, s/n/hf/g, scalp, neck, hands, feet, genitalia; face-mm, f/e/e/n/l, face, ears, eyelids, nose, lips, mucous membrane; mal, malignant; Rpr, repair; s/n/agen/trk, scalp, neck, axillae, external genitalia, trunk and/or extremities (including hands and feet).

reimbursement from insurance and patients. There are additional expenses that a physician incurs (**Box 2**). With inflation, the price of many of these items increases yearly. Some expenses, such as surgical tables or lasers, are depreciated over a period of years, whereas supplies are counted at the time of purchase. A skilled accountant can help minimize your tax burden.

A physician starting a practice needs to calculate projected expenses and determine how many patients they need to see based on insurance rates and visit/procedure type in order to break even. There are efficiencies with economies of scale, where above a certain amount of fixed expense there is more profit. Seeing one extra patient per hour if it does not markedly change the cost of support staff, supplies, and other costs can be an important way to boost income, especially as physicians become more efficient in their practice. However, there are balancing measures, as a busier physician often needs more staff resources. In addition, if patients are waiting longer to be seen, cannot get appointments in a timely manner, or feel rushed in their visit, they may be unhappy with care and less likely to refer new patients to the practice. If the physician sees more patients but then spends more time charting after hours, that may be an unacceptable increase in daily workload relative to income.

For a physician who is given an employment offer, there will typically be an expectation of the number of patients per hour (eg, 4 per hour), and/or RVU goal. If the physician is given a base salary (or hourly rate), this has been calculated based on the practice of estimating what they will be able to collect from insurance and patients for the physician services. If the wRVU threshold is the 50th percentile (for example, 7329 per year), and the average dermatology encounter yields 1.49 wRVU, a physician needs to see 4919 patients per year. Assume for simplicity that this is only outpatient, and at a large group will provide 3 weeks of vacation, 1 week of CME, and 1 week of sick time, for a total of 47 weeks per year for 4919 wRVU divided by 47 wk/y = 106 patients per week. Therefore, you see 27 patients per day, 4 days per week, correct? Well, you have to account for no-shows, which may be 10% in a small practice but 25% to 50% in a large academic center. Hence, schedules often are overbooked, or appointment slots are very short to account for no-shows to yield an end-of-day appropriate number of patients to generate enough revenue long term.

Physicians employed by large groups and academic centers are not immune to productivity targets and ever-increasing demands to see more patients. A firm grasp on coding will help physicians be paid appropriately for the work they already perform. Being comfortable and efficient with procedures is helpful. Delegating nonphysician tasks to others can increase productivity (initial patient history, charting, photographs, obtaining biopsy supplies, filling out pathology paperwork, placing laboratory orders, calling back patients with normal laboratory results, refill requests, prior authorizations). Optimizing the amount of work that physicians do that is directly related to patient care may also help improve job satisfaction and reduce physician burnout, which can increase career longevity and overall lifetime earnings. Be aware that studies show female physicians are often expected by patients to spend more time with them in the visit, and that female physicians report more burnout.[25]

## DISCUSSION
### Section 3: Value Beyond Direct Profits

Even the most financially savvy dermatologist convinced of their ability to start a solo practice and become successful should consider other aspects of a practice/job to determine the right fit. Recall in Section 1, taking time to envision what your ideal practice would look like, considering aspects such as practice setting, type of work, location, days per week, hours per day. In addition, you should consider time off, patient load, income and expenses, and other factors (**Box 3**). Is it worth spending an extra hour a day in card to earn more money or is the time better spent with family or hiking in a forest? You must make these choices.

Also, consider that some of these benefits may not be as simple as "yes it is offered." For example, although a paid maternity leave of 6 to 8 weeks may be a benefit at larger institutions/groups and other groups may provide FMLA-mandated leave of up to 12 weeks, this often just protects your job and is unpaid. In solo practice or small group private practice, the offered leave time may differ from what you feel comfortable taking (consider if you need to pay overhead while on leave or if you will lose patients or other aspects of your practice that you have built up during leave). State or private short-term disability to replace a portion of the income may be available, but it has income limits that are still lower than an expected dermatologist salary.

As you can see, there are many aspects of a job offer or starting one's own practice that should be considered apart from just the salary.

## SUMMARY
### Section 4: Putting It Together and Building Your Own Adaptive Mathematical Model

So how do you take all of this information to estimate your own profitability? Does it seem a little intimidating? Don't be afraid. You don't have to make your own model from scratch. We did it for you.

Although this article aims to provide you an understanding of CPT coding and variations in insurance payment, your primary focus should be assessing your own productivity expectations, targets, bonus thresholds, and comparison to your peers locally and nationally. Try to track your own productivity and periodically meet with practice managers to assess your performance and look for ways to improve these measures. This may include auditing charts to see if billing is optimized, adding more visits to the schedule, adding support staff, adding new services, additional marketing, and so forth.

You can use these 2 tables to estimate your own value/productivity (**Table 4**) and then compare profitability in different practice settings (**Table 5**), both available as an editable file to download online. **Table 4** offers a basic outline of how to calculate your profitability and potential earnings. It can be modified for your particular practice (many procedure codes may not be relevant for the general dermatologist), but the most important thing is to be realistic with yourself in estimating how many CPT codes you expect to bill in 1 day.

We have populated **Table 4** with Medicare reimbursement national averages for 2023, but this can be easily adjusted for future years and catered to your locale by using the Medicare Physician Free Schedule Tool (**Fig. 2**). In addition, if you anticipate that the private insurance of most patients seen at your practice pays a multiplier of Medicare (eg, 1.2×), this can be input in Column J to give you a closer estimate of potential earnings. If your employer bases salary off of wRVUs, this information is available in hidden column H. Note that for many codes, if performing more than one on a single given patient in one visit (ie, 3 separate malignant excisions on the back of one patient), the first should be placed in column L (SOLO) and the rest in column M (MULTI).

Your final annual estimated collections will depend on how many days a week you work and how many weeks of vacation you take. Once you populate your collections estimate, you can then use it in Row 2 of **Table 5** to help compare different offers.

## Section 5: Examples

Now let's compare some offers! You have 3 jobs offers available to you. We will assume for this exercise that you estimate to be able generate $800,000/y in revenue. The first (job 1) is at an academic institution that offers a base salary of

**Table 5**
**Compare profitability in different practice settings**

| Job Offer | Job 1 | Job 2 | Job 3 |
|---|---|---|---|
| Your collections | | | |
| Percentage of collections (your piece of the pie) | | | |
| Your earnings | | | |
| Base salary? | | | |
| Med Mal (+ if THEY pay; − if YOU pay) | | | |
| Health Ins (+ if THEY pay; otherwise, your share [−]) | | | |
| License/DEA/CME | | | |
| Auto allowance | | | |
| Retirement[a] | | | |
| Retirement match | | | |
| Other | | | |
| Other | | | |
| "Actual" compensation[b] | | | |

[a] Very variable. For this, assume any retirement you want for lean is out of your pocket (not in formula, as self-contribution is taken from earnings/base salary). Generous employer lets you shelter 5% and matches 5%. 2023 employer + employee maximum contribution is $66,000.
[b] Minus state and federal tax.
*Abbreviations:* DEA, Drug Enforcement Administration.

$325,000 with no dependency on collections; the second (job 2) is a large private equity group that offers 50% collections, and the third (job 3) is a private practice office that offers 40% collections. (Keep in mind that many nonacademic contracts provide a first-year salary guarantee and then switch to payment based fully on collections after 1–2 years).

Although at first glance it may appear that the second job is the best offer, we must think about all potential costs and benefits (**Table 6**). If we consider health insurance, medical malpractice, and retirement matching, job 3 now comes out on top if considering earnings alone. Nevertheless, perhaps you value more vacation time, less call time, or the option of seeing fewer patients per hour? Then, maybe job 1 now seems the most appealing.

You must also consider how much freedom each choice gives you. For example, in job 1 and 2, vacations or other time off must often be scheduled many months in advance, whereas choice 3 may be much more flexible. You must also consider how much influence you have over your employees; choice 3 usually allows input for firing and hiring of personnel that best suit you. Do not

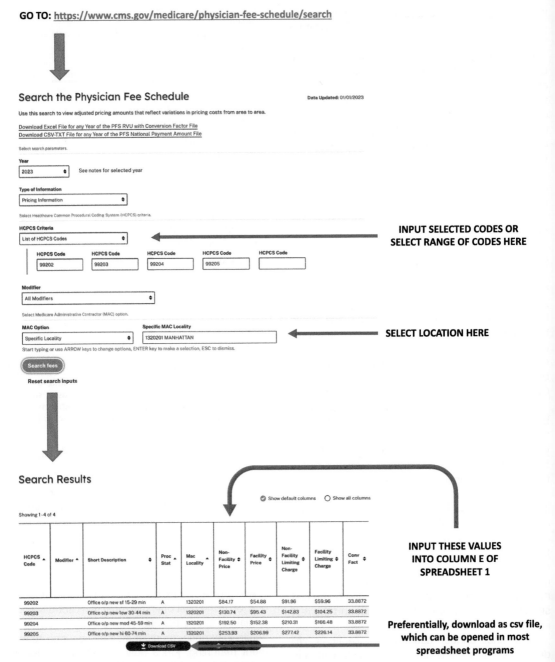

**Fig. 2.** How to use the Physician Fee Schedule Tool.

forget noncompete agreements, which all positions will have. These can be geographically calculated from ANY location at which the practice has a presence. Some larger groups may cover the whole state! Although these are currently under review at the federal level, do not count on them going away any time soon. Finally, do not fool yourself and say I will only take this great paying job for a few years to pay off my debts them move on. Life happens in the

interim, and later, selling a house and uprooting a spouse and children become very difficult. Try and make your first choice your final one.

As you can see, although our basic formula (Profit = Revenue – Expenses) is necessary to understand how we make money in dermatology, your final take-home salary should consider an evaluation of all the potential costs and benefits available. We encourage you to use this article

**Table 6**
**Comparing offers example**

| Job Offer: | Job 1 | Job 2 | Job 3 |
|---|---|---|---|
| Your collections | $800,000.00 | $800,000.00 | $800,000.00 |
| Percentage of collections (your piece of the pie) | 0 | 50 | 40 |
| Your earnings | $0.00 | $400,000.00 | $320,000.00 |
| Base salary? | $325,000.00 | $0.00 | $0.00 |
| Med mal (+ if THEY pay; − if YOU pay) | $10,500.00 | −$10,500.00 | $10,500.00 |
| Health ins (+ if THEY pay; otherwise, your share [−]) | $14,500.00 | −$14,500.00 | $14,500.00 |
| License/DEA/CME | $1000.00 | −$1000.00 | $1000.00 |
| Auto allowance | $0.00 | $0.00 | $1000.00 |
| Retirement[a] | $22,500.00 | $22,500.00 | $22,500.00 |
| Retirement match | $22,500.00 | $0.00 | $43,500.00 |
| Vacation time | 5 wk | 3 wk | 3 wk |
| Call responsibilities | No | Yes | Yes |
| "Actual" compensation[b] | $373,500.00 | $374,000.00 | $390,500.00 |

[a] Very variable. For this, assume any retirement you want for lean is out of your pocket (not in formula as self-contribution taken from earnings/base salary). Generous employer lets you shelter 5% and matches 5%. 2023 employer + employee maximum contribution is $66,000.
[b] Minus state and federal tax.

and the tools provided to examine your potential earnings holistically to help better assess your future profitability.

## CLINICS CARE POINTS

- Look before you leap.
- Money isnt everything. Happiness might be.
- Assess you own effieiciency and be sure if messhes with both your own financial goals and visin of your practice.
- Don't get mad. Get data.

## DISCLOSURE

Dr K.M. Derrick, Dr N.M. Golbari, and Dr D.M. Siegel have no relevant disclosures.

## REFERENCES

1. Fees & Insurance. Oregon Coast Dermatology. Available at: http://www.oregonderm.com/fees-insurance/. Accessed December 20, 2022.
2. Margosian E. Cash Only. Dermatology World 2018; 40–4. Available at: http://digitaleditions.walsworthprintgroup.com/publication/?i=482834&article_id=3036738&view=articleBrowser.
3. Lewis M. How do doctors get paid? Ideal Medical Practices. Available at: https://idealmedicalpractices.typepad.com/ideal_medical_practices/2009/02/how-do-doctors-get-paid-.html. Published February 21, 2009. Accessed December 20, 2022.
4. Coding Resource Center. American Academy of Dermatology. Available at: https://www.aad.org/member/practice/coding. Accessed January 12, 2023.
5. Miller A. Cracking the Code: Evaluation and Management in 2021. Dermatology World 2022;22–3. http://digitaleditions.walsworthprintgroup.com/publication/?m=12468&i=678355&p=18&ver=html5.
6. CPT QuickRef. Version 4.3.2. American Medical Association; 2022. Available at: https://apps.apple.com/us/app/cpt-quickref/id426712025.
7. Medicare Fee Schedule. American Academy of Dermatology. Available at: https://www.aad.org/member/practice/mips/fee-schedule. Accessed December 20, 2022.
8. 0108-facility versus non-facility reimbursement: Incorrect coding. CMS.gov. Available at: https://www.cms.gov/Research-Statistics-Data-and-Systems/Monitoring-Programs/Medicare-FFS-Compliance-Programs/Recovery-Audit-Program/Approved-RAC-Topics-Items/0108-Facility-vs-Non-Facility-Reimbursement. Published October 1, 2018. Accessed December 20, 2022.
9. CMS updates Medicare conversion factor; new fee schedule expected soon. California Medical Association. Available at: https://www.cmadocs.org/newsroom/news/view/ArticleId/50010/CMS-updates-Medicare-conversion-factor-New-fee-schedule-expected-soon.

Published January 11, 2023. Accessed January 12, 2023.

10. Physician fee schedule look-up tol. CMS. Available at: https://www.cms.gov/Medicare/Medicare-Fee-for-Service-Payment/PFSlookup. Accessed January 12, 2023.

11. Calculating Medicare fee schedule rates. Available at: https://www.asha.org/practice/reimbursement/medicare/calculating-medicare-fee-schedule-rates/. Accessed December 20, 2022.

12. Procedure price lookup for outpatient services. Medicare.gov. Available at: https://www.medicare.gov/procedure-price-lookup/. Accessed December 20, 2022.

13. Eastern J. Dermatology: The Last Refuge for Private Practice? Cutis 2014;94(3):117–8.

14. Kaplan DA. Group purchasing: Save Money by aligning with other physicians. Medical Economics. Available at: https://www.medicaleconomics.com/view/group-purchasing-save-money-aligning-other-physicians. Published November 12, 2020. Accessed December 20, 2022.

15. Lopez E, Neuman T, Jacobson G, Levitt L. How much more than Medicare do private insurers pay? A review of the literature. Available at: https://www.kff.org/medicare/issue-brief/how-much-more-than-medicare-do-private-insurers-pay-a-review-of-the-literature/. Published May 1, 2020. Accessed December 20, 2022.

16. Gooch K. 74% of physicians are hospital or corporate employees, with pandemic fueling increase. Becker's Hospital Review. Available at: https://www.beckershospitalreview.com/hospital-physician-relationships/74-of-physicians-are-hospital-or-corporate-employees-with-pandemic-fueling-increase.html. Published April 19, 2022. Accessed December 20, 2022.

17. Fighting Medicare payment cuts in 2023 and beyond. American Academy of Dermatology. Available at: https://www.aad.org/member/publications/impact/2022-issue-3/fighting-medicare-payment-cuts-2023. Accessed December 20, 2022.

18. O'Reilly KB. Medicare physician pay cuts underscore need to fix broken system. American Medical Association. Available at: https://www.ama-assn.org/practice-management/medicare-medicaid/medicare-physician-pay-cuts-underscore-need-fix-broken-system. Published December 20, 2022. Accessed December 20, 2022.

19. Creadore A, Desai S, Li SJ, et al. Insurance acceptance, appointment wait time, and dermatologist access across practice types in the US. JAMA Dermatology 2021;157(2):181. https://doi.org/10.1001/jamadermatol.2020.5173.

20. Medicaid-to-medicare fee index. Available at: https://www.kff.org/medicaid/state-indicator/medicaid-to-medicare-fee-index/?currentTimeframe=0&sortModel=%7B%22colId%22%3A%22Location%22%2C%22sort%22%3A%22asc%22%7D. Published June 22, 2022. Accessed December 20, 2022.

21. Physician Manual. eMedNY.org. Available at: https://www.emedny.org/ProviderManuals/Physician/index.aspx. Accessed December 20, 2022.

22. Understanding RVU compensation. William Sullivan, Attorney at Law. Available at: https://sullivanlegal.us/understanding-rvu-compensation/. Published June 4, 2022. Accessed December 20, 2022.

23. Staff Compensation. Medical Group Management Association. Available at: https://www.mgma.com/data/participate-in-benchmarking-surveys/resources-for-compensation-and-production-survey/2022-mgma-datadive-compensation-and-production-sur/view-all. Accessed January 10, 2023.

24. 2021 Annual Physician Compensation Survey. Available at: https://www.phg.com/wp-content/uploads/2022/04/2021-Physician-Compensation-Report_-updated-0821.pdf. Published 2021. Accessed January 12, 2023.

25. Yeluru H, Newton HL, Kapoor R. Physician Burnout Through the Female Lens: A Silent Crisis. Front Public Health 2022;10:880061.

# Private Equity: the Good

Barry Leshin, MD

## KEYWORDS

• Dermatology • Practice management • Private equity

## KEY POINTS

- Private equity backed dermatology practice management companies (DPM) provide a viable practice model that merits consideration as a pathway to successful professional and practice development.
- Dermatology-specific management expertise can be deployed to enhance a practice's operations and profitability while providing an environment of professional satisfaction and high-quality patient care.
- The advent of DPM has triggered some controversy within the specialty, which is discussed herein.

## PRACTICE MODELS

There are several practice models that have long been employed in dermatology. These models have served us well, appealing to a variety of personal and professional goals.

### Solo Practice

Solo practice has long been popular for dermatologists. As an outpatient specialty independent of the ancillary services provided by a medical center, such a practice can be appealing to individuals who by nature are self-reliant, and desire complete autonomy and the satisfaction of operating a medical practice. Such an approach permits the achievement of financial or reputational success by one's own hand. There are some disadvantages. Capital expenses on supplies, instruments and equipment, and navigation of ever changing medical, technologic, regulatory and reporting environments can be onerous. The inherent absence of direct collegial relationships and internal peer review can present challenges to remaining current and knowledgeable in the field. Time away from the practice due to vacation or illness can have an enormous impact on income. Exiting

practice can be difficult. Finding a successor may not be possible, in which case, the practice's patients must be notified, and the practice's hard assets sold.

### Dermatology Group Practice

Partnering with other dermatologists with aligned practice goals has evolved into a popular model. Sharing the cost of resources such as space, equipment, supplies, capital expenses, staff, legal, revenue cycle management and accounting costs, and marketing is vital in controlling ever-increasing overhead, particularly with rising inflation and for fixed costs unrelated to number of providers. The size of the practice affords a degree of leverage when negotiating supply and equipment costs, and to some extent in the negotiation of reimbursement rates with various payers. Group size also permits employment of staff with specialized skills to meet the demands of practice management in an increasingly complex environment. Multiple providers afford an opportunity for flexibility in schedules, cross-coverage for major life events and succession planning. As mentioned

The author has practiced six years affiliated with a dermatology practice management company.
125 New Castle Drive, Chapel Hill, NC 27517, USA
E-mail address: barry.leshin@yahoo.com

Dermatol Clin 41 (2023) 589–596
https://doi.org/10.1016/j.det.2023.04.003

derm.theclinics.com

above, internal peer review affords a safety net in meeting ever-evolving standards of care.

## Multispecialty Group

In addition to the many advantages described in dermatology group practice, a multispecialty group creates an environment with internally referred patients, and ready access to colleagues in other disciplines. This model can be attractive to patients seeking all their care under a single roof. There is some risk of being marginalized by our small specialty size, but also opportunity derived from strong patient demand for dermatology services.

## Academic

The traditional academic model of medical practice affords the many advantages of the large multispecialty group practice, with the additional attraction to participate in the education of medical students and training of residents, to conduct meaningful research, and to enjoy the prestige and unique opportunities associated with this setting. There are challenges to practicing in such an environment. Compensation may be lower, so that the academic missions of teaching and research can be financially supported. There may be a complex institutional bureaucracy, disruptive leadership changes at the senior or departmental level, and the agendas of new leaders may not be aligned with your personal goals. Finally, practice development may be hampered by competing demands for teaching and research, and by difficult patient access in a confusing campus with inherent challenges of traffic and parking, especially for our elderly patients.

## DERMATOLOGY PRACTICE MANAGEMENT (DPM) COMPANY

The objective of this article is not to fully describe the many nuances in the practice models mentioned above, but rather to focus on the private equity backed dermatology practice management company. There are numerous features that have triggered the interest of private equity in the specialty of dermatology. The specialty is highly fragmented, with extensive redundancies in overhead across providers. Additionally, there is a manpower shortage in dermatology, a skin cancer epidemic and an aging population resulting in a great demand for medical, surgical and cosmetic services. Our intent is to describe in greater depth the many appealing features of this model, and to address some of the controversy that has been generated as the model has gained ground by attracting 15% of practicing dermatologists.[1–3]

The DPM management team is composed of a highly specialized workforce with expertise in the many phases of medical practice management, and specifically dermatology practice management. The sophistication, acumen, and breadth of specialty-specific management expertise of such a high level is not generally available or affordable in the typically sized dermatology group. The primary elements of a DPM, which will be described in some depth, include operations, financial management, information technology, and human resources. It is important to have some understanding of the breadth and the complexity of practice management to appreciate the critical need for dedicated expert resources to provide comprehensive support. Doctors are enabled to focus on what they are trained to do, which is to take care of patients, and to leave the complexity of practice management in the hands of those with specialized expertise. While many multi-specialty group practices and academic centers have large management teams, the dermatology-specific expertise adds an enormous dimension and value to all employees.

## Operations

There are many essential ingredients in operational management.

### Compliance management

All practices have regulatory requirements. The onerous reporting demands of MIPS and MACRA requires ongoing supervision, as does adherence to established governmental regulations of HIPAA and CLIA. All of these require regular monitoring, adjustments to changes in reporting requirements, and an understanding of key elements that are targets for external audits. Billing and coding is an everchanging soup of regulations, and providers must continually be educated and monitored for adherence to rigorous documentation of patient encounters. Regulations for supervision of non-physician providers, usually stipulated at the state level by medical boards, also require policies and procedures and ongoing monitoring.

### Payer contract negotiations and network management

DPMs with numerous providers covering a large catchment area can enable payers in filling panels, including coverage for lower density areas and with negotiation of reimbursement rates. Excellent aggregated data on such matters as revenue per visit, support staff cost per visit, supply cost per visit is meaningful for payers (and will be meaningful as the 'value-base' paradigm matures). Using centralized and sophisticated revenue cycle management for a large group of providers streamlines payers' processes and provides value for them. Providing quality data and information such as identifying that the group's Mohs surgeons are fellowship-trained and demonstrating surgeons' metrics such as number layers/case, and percentage of cases that cancers are on the head and neck vs trunk, extremities.

## Facility and supplies management
Interruptions in patient care due to facility issues, e.g., HVAC, leaky roof, plumbing, electricity, can be costly and frustrating for patients and providers alike. An ability to efficiently diagnose problems and mobilize necessary resources moves a huge burden to trained operations management. In short, a DPM has a greater breadth of human resources, and this permits a more focused approach to facility management. Similarly, interruptions in supplies can bring clinical activity to a halt. Monitoring supply chains for potential downstream interruptions can prevent such occurrences. The scale of practice permits sharing of supplies across practice sites, and direct coordination with suppliers mitigates disruptions. For example, the current lidocaine shortage affects everyone, but the larger group size proves advantageous with vendors. Also, lidocaine allocation can be adjusted across a panel of providers and sites depending on need/usage.

## Lab operations
Supply chain, equipment maintenance and emergency service, and staffing issues can interrupt laboratory workflow, and hamper delivery of care. Proactively monitoring supplies and service/maintenance contracts can help avoid unpleasant surprises, and efficient cross training of staff across multiple practice sites can circumvent staffing disruptions. Also, professional management ensures that a laboratory is always prepared for CLIA inspection. Larger practices can support larger labs where more sophisticated testing and coordinated care can provide providers additional benefit and collaboration.

## Development of new practice sites
Opportunities to grow a practice with the addition of a new practice site requires significant effort. Reviewing population demographics, competition, demand for services, availability of adequate facility, providers and staff are critical to any de novo practice site. The financial analysis of return on investment and time to positive cash flow are pivotal to the decision to deploy capital, which is funded by the PE investors rather than one's personal resources. Finally, the integration of a new practice includes a significant effort in readying office space and training staff.

## Development of new service lines
Like new practice sites, critical pro forma analysis is essential to successful deployment of capital for new service lines. Understanding practice demographics, unmet demand, marketing, space and staffing issues and time to ramp up volume to achieve profitability are essential undertakings before capital expenditure is deemed worthwhile.

## Marketing
Marketing efforts have evolved from primarily traditional print media and hardcopy mailings to social media and search engine optimization. Specialized expertise in this area adds great value to creating a practice's public profile and generating demand.

## Crisis management
We exist in an era of devastation from floods, hurricanes, tornadoes, and fires which can cause extraordinary property damage to medical office buildings. Firearms are a menace in our society and shooting tragedies occur with a staggering frequency. Our recent experience with the COVID-19 pandemic demonstrated how a centralized approach by a clinical governance council working in harmony with the management team could establish safety policies and operational protocols to benefit the patients and the many individual practices who otherwise would have faced this medical and financial threat in isolation. The very real potential for serious illness and death required a thoughtful approach to protecting patients and staff. Introduction of work furloughs and scheduling cutbacks were complex human resource decisions, while preserving staff job security and benefits was extraordinarily challenging. For instance, at the physician level, base compensation was lowered (not total compensation), protecting the DPM's cash flow. While there was brief suspension of 401(k), full benefits were otherwise maintained even for furloughed staff. The crisis team kept staff and providers current on CDC recommendations and individual state guidelines, the clinical implications for practices, and established criteria for what kind of Mohs cases could be scheduled. All clinical practitioners uniformly expressed gratitude for the oversight and guidance provided by the physician and management leadership during the pandemic.

## Financial Management

### Accounting, taxes, financial planning and analysis

Financial management of a practice begins with extraordinary detail in accounting matters. While tax returns and audit remain the province of certified public accountants, the minute details of monitoring balance sheets, profit and loss statements, revenue and expenses is fundamental. Expertise in development of annual budgets, monitoring for deviations, and rigorous analysis of financial data permits successful planning and comparison with industry benchmarks. Tracking of practice profitability requires reviewing metrics like visit volumes, workdays, revenue/visit and support hours/visit. Cyclical seasonal revenue lags must be evaluated and anticipated so that expenses can be budgeted accordingly. Medical practices are susceptible to embezzlement and establishing strict and comprehensive safeguards for oversight of cash transactions is critical.

### State and legal reporting

State taxing agencies require extensive reporting for income tax withholding, corporate taxes, sales and use tax, and unemployment insurance tax, and for provider license fees.

### Revenue cycle management

Revenue cycle management is complex and requires attention to multiple key steps to ensure payment for services in a timely manner. These steps include: (1) Patient registration, including accuracy in date entry, insurance verification and coordination of benefits for patients with multiple policies; (2) documentation in the medical record supports billing (CPT) codes, and that payer guidelines for claims are met; (3) accurate claim entry into the medical billing software, into an intermediary clearinghouse, and management of rejected claims; (4) claim status follow up; (5) review of payer remittance advice; (6) resolution/appeal of claim denials; (7) posting of payments into billing software; (8) mailing statements to patients for balances owed. Measuring performance is integral to evaluating performance of RCM, and parameters include aging of accounts receivable, collection of copays due, and percentage of allowable charges collected.

### Accounts payable

As in any business, short term debt due to routine expenses are accrued. In a typical medical practice, these expenses would include medical and non-medical equipment and supplies, and utilities. Rigorous attention to bookkeeping details that reconciles vendor invoices and payment is essential to the financial health of the practice.

### Capital for growth

Medical practice growth, be it expansion to a new practice site or addition of new service lines can require significant capital. Additionally, capital is also necessary for office space renovation, new equipment, e.g., lasers, recruitment of and payment to new providers before collections ramp up, and computers and software. Decisions to raise and/or deploy capital through cash flow, equity, debt or capital calls require sophistication, experience and expertise beyond that of a typical physician.

## Information Technology (IT)

### Electronic health records

EHRs are an essential component of healthcare information technology, and in current use, integrate the health record, scheduling, and billing and collection functions. Given the breadth of importance in these key areas, the role of expertise in IT is critical in selecting, integrating, and operating the vital software and hardware. Dermatology-specific EHRs have made integration into workflow and user training less of an obstacle, but ongoing support in maintaining operability, privacy and network security requires special expertise. Linkage of important health record data fields with professional society databases (such as the American Academy of Dermatology's DataDerm)) must meet MIPS/MACRA regulatory requirements and support societies' research and advocacy functions. Additionally, EHR vendors often offer enhanced pricing based on the size and scale of group.

### Help desk

Under the auspices of an internally based support system (help desk), the uniformity of software and hardware across myriad users permits prompt resolution of hardware and software problems and minimizes workflow disruption on both the patient care and administrative function of a busy practice.

### Phone system support

Telephony remains a key interface for practice operations. The capacity to manage inbound and outbound calls with patients for scheduling, billing inquiries, and for direct contact with nursing and providers must be HIPAA compliant and robust. Integrated into system support includes incorporation of queueing and automatic call overflow management for peak call hours to enhance efficiency and patient satisfaction. Secure after hour messaging and paging systems are vital for patient safety and must be tailored for providers' preferences.

### Website management
Surveys regularly demonstrate that patients desire web face interface with their medical providers. The digital strategy must be ethical, professional, secure, easy to navigate, and seamlessly interface with the practice's electronic health record, scheduling, and billing software, and permit online registration. The website should also include key business information such as location with navigation, spectrum of services provided, useful information about such services, insurances accepted, and provider profiles.

### Proprietary practice analytics
Part of the drive for practice consolidation comes from a shift toward value-based healthcare, where physicians are compensated for keeping patients healthy, in place of the traditional fee-for-service model. As noted above, comprehensive data analysis is pivotal in contract negotiations, and in confirming that payers are paying per contract on all charge submissions. Additionally, practice management software permits aggregation of cost data that can serve to strengthen the practice's negotiation of rates with payers.

### Network security
Breeches of security in a practice's network have profound implications for patients, and penalties can be devastating. Sophisticated monitoring and rapid intervention are paramount. Many small practices do not have the expertise or the budget to implement sophisticated security measures and testing.

## Human Resources

### Recruiting/training
Employee turnover is integral to today's workplace. Taking advantage of internet services and agencies is essential and is a multistep process. Screening applicant qualifications and work history, telephone, video and in person interviews, and follow up conversations with references requires allocation of time and interpersonal skills. Successful integration of new employees requires intensive training in policies and procedures of the practice in addition to the actual job training itself.

### Employee benefits
A comprehensive benefit plan is vital to employee recruitment and retention. DPMs are of a size that diversify the risk pool for insurers, allowing for some advantage in rates. Administration of health, dental, vision, disability, and life insurance, and flexible spending accounts, retirement plans and payroll are frequently outsourced to a third-party company, while the human resource manager serves in the key role of being the interface between that company and employees. Integral to management of this benefit structure is the annual negotiation with health insurers to achieve an optimal rate and benefit structure, and a subsequent intensive review of options with employees during the enrollment period.

### Employee agreements
For nursing and administrative staff and new providers, an HR manager maintains up-to-date job descriptions and expectations, and establishment of an efficient hierarchy, discipline and reporting structure.

### Employee relations
A happy staff is a productive one, and given the time and money required to recruit and train new employees much can be done to enhance job satisfaction. Key to this is open and regular communication in the form of thorough performance and job satisfaction reviews. In times of employee crisis, establishment of an internal non-profit agency with 501(c)3 status provides an avenue for contributions by staff to a pool of emergency use funds to allocate according to need.

## WHAT ACCOUNTS FOR THE SUCCESS OF INVESTOR BACKED DPM?

Dermatology has a tradition of many solo practitioners and small group practices. The practices have operated successfully as silos, and the value of independence and total control has resonated for many dermatologists. The DPM model alternatively succeeds through the consolidation of these silos, elimination of expensive redundancies in staffing, equipment, and supplies, and by leveraging expertise in cost education with payers and vendors. An additional core advantage offered by DPMs is the breadth and depth of expertise deployed to address the onerous administrative burden of managing a practice in an era of increasing practice overhead and declining reimbursement, and the veil of regulatory challenges.

There is some similarity of drivers that bring physicians to consider affiliation. Selection of a DPM that understands the importance to physicians of maintaining the highest standards of patient care and a patient-centric culture can enhance the joy of practice. The vetting of a company requires a thorough, thoughtful, multipronged approach, and can be fraught with potholes. Of greatest importance in determining if the company is a good fit is communication with colleagues who are practicing under a DPM's umbrella.

## OTHER DRIVERS THAT MAKE THE DPM MODEL WORTHY OF CONSIDERATION:
### Geographic

Finding an opportunity in a specific geographic area can be challenging. Finding the right fit includes consideration of issues such as where does one's family live, what work opportunities are available for both you and your spouse, what is the cost of living, what is the housing market, how are the schools, and what are the cultural and recreational offerings. DPMs are flourishing in almost all regions of the country and are usually interested in adding providers. And if you are looking for a de novo startup opportunity in an unserved area, many DPMs are prepared to capitalize establishment of a new practice.

### Group Infrastructure

DPMs not only provide the dermatology-specific administrative personnel and the capital support for integration of a new physician, but also an established group of peers-colleagues. Subspecialized providers in Mohs surgery, cosmetic practice, and dermatopathology may serve as mentors and enhance one's practice. If you have specialized training or a particular area of interest, the group environment of a DPM can provide a willing source of patient referral as new providers are vetted by existing partners to ensure a good fit and quality mindset.

### Ready Capital

Most successful practices eye opportunities for growth. Such growth may be in the form of addition of new providers to meet patient demand, purchase of new devices, establishment of new service lines and practice sites. There is an ever present need to stay current with hardware and software upgrades. DPMs expertly analyze investment opportunities to enhance their practices and are prepared to deploy capital accordingly.

### Equity

Many DPMs offer equity opportunity to providers, uniquely aligning incentives amongst clinicians, the management team and financial sponsors. Joining a group of like-minded colleagues focused on the success of the enterprise can offer financial return by delivering fair market value for their practice should there be a change in ownership of the DPM. Additionally, the ownership participation in a DPM which includes multiple practices and multiple practice sites affords more diversification of risk than other models.

### Eliminate Administrative Burden

As mentioned previously, the administration of medical practice in an era of increasing overhead, declining reimbursement, and regulatory challenges can be a burden, affecting quality of life and leading to burnout.

### Exit Strategy and Succession Planning

Mid and late career physicians are often frustrated in development of a retirement strategy. Questions of continued care of a practice's patients, continued employment of staff, and future lease or purchase of space are primary considerations. Recruitment and integration of a new provider can be challenging, particularly as newer graduates saddled with educational debt are less willing and able to contemplate practice purchase. The DPM is able to offer a guaranteed salary for the first year, and a subsequent production-based compensation plan mirroring that offered to dermatologists in other models. Sale of a practice to another physician or to a health care conglomerate is typically based on the purchase of equipment, supplies and accounts receivable. The value of a career devoted to developing and nurturing a successful highly regarded medical practice is completely discounted in this era in which intangible goodwill has no monetary value.

### Improve Efficiency

Patient scheduling, space utilization, appropriate staffing/support, and administrative workflow are vital not only to profitability but also to provider, staff and patient satisfaction. Thoughtful and expert review and analysis can provide practical and sustainable improvement in efficiencies and can mitigate physician burnout.

### Physician Leadership

Physician leadership of a DPM has a primary responsibility to establish uniform quality, safety and patient service standards across the entire practice, which should be explicitly recognized by management. Opportunities exist to contribute to clinical governance through experience and expertise, outside of traditional academic models.

### Vetting of New Practices, Providers by Colleagues

Physicians have a keen insight into quality of practices joining the group, and management should include rigorous professional review of practices being considered for partnership.

## Surveys of Patients and Staff

A patient-centric practice culture is the expressed goal of most practices. Patient satisfaction is a key component. It is essential that survey instruments are expertly developed, regularly distributed to patients, and that the results of the survey are scrutinized and acted upon as necessary. Staff opinions of the workplace regarding employment issues, provider performance, and patient safety work to enhance a practice's quality, and engagement of staff in this way expresses appreciation by acknowledging their voice and ascribing value to such feedback.

## Prevent Burnout

Physician burnout is real and is appropriately receiving close study. Administrative responsibilities, bureaucratic regulatory demands, electronic health records are regularly cited as precipitating factors. A successful DPM can promote physician wellbeing and fulfillment by attending to an organizational culture of administrative and physician co-leadership, professionalism, teamwork, and flexibility.[4,5]

## CONTROVERSIES

It is important to understand the mechanics of the industry. A private equity company will purchase (usually with loans and capital from limited partners) and consolidate multiple practices into a single company, which represents one of many companies in its portfolio. The private equity firm collects from its investors 1-2% of transaction costs and expects roughly 20% return on the investment after paying interest on its debt. (As interest rates rise, private equity companies will be much more selective in their acquisitions, and in general practice valuations will decline.) Revenue is enhanced and overhead is decreased via the deployment of a management team's expertise focused on utilizing scale to streamline operational efficiencies. Within a period of 3 to 7 years, the successful company is sold to another investor looking to consolidate with other similar companies. Physician practice owners who have assumed risk by affiliation with a DPM may receive equity in the company as part of the transaction, and in return can earn multiples of invested capital. The guardrail of business investment is the inherent risk-reward calculus. In the case of investor backed DPMs, the risk of competition creating unsustainable valuation multiples, and the risk of increasing interest rates in highly leveraged transactions add traction to the risk-reward equation faced by investors and aligned physicians.

Many authors and pundits have suggested that private equity backed DPMs pose a threat to physician autonomy and clinical decision making. State medical boards address the corporatization of medicine through regulatory requirements that prioritize physician control over all clinical decisions and judgment. Despite this, the concerns of many physicians considering the DPM model are consistent: Will the company exert full control of my schedule and determine the number and types of patients I see? Is my staff's employment at risk? Will my compensation and benefits suffer? Will I need to meet quotas for biopsies and cryo-surgeries? Will I be required to supervise too many mid-level providers? Indeed, such unfortunate characteristics have been highlighted in the lay press. [Who among us has not witnessed a newspaper that is prepared to sensationalize unprofessional behavior and ascribe it broadly and indiscriminately?] Will I be forced to use the company's pathology services and Mohs surgeon, or will I have discretion over referrals?

Given its fiduciary responsibility to investors, the DPM is often ascribed numerous nefarious qualities as it strives to achieve profitability. Acknowledging that the DPM is highly motivated to operate a profitable enterprise, the best ones achieve this by nurturing a content clinical and administrative support staff and partnering with a physician workforce aligned with and conducive to its growth, thereby creating an attractiveness for subsequent acquisition. Moreover, scrutiny by regulatory agencies and by its competition are compelling factors for operational transparency. It is essential that the company protects its investment against risk. Healthcare is highly regulated, and strict adherence is vital so that costly penalties for violations are avoided. Another key risk is disenfranchisement of the physician workforce. Alignment of financial interests, an enhanced work environment without administrative stress, and thoughtfully developed guidelines for operational policies and procedures are motivating forces that nullify claims of egregious behavior.

Multiple articles have posited that private equity backed DPMs are responsible for increased spending for dermatology care via overutilization of mid-level providers, and unnecessary procedures, and that the misalignment of incentives with value-based care have compromised patient outcomes.[1,2,6] However, one recent analysis concluded that private equity DPMs had little impact on health care spending, with modest increases in patient volumes per dermatologist and slightly higher reimbursement, consistent with a model that removes impediments to efficiency and leverages scale[7] These concerns and suppositions, and many others, deserve the methodical study and analysis warranted by any new practice model, including not only private equity backed DPMs, but also the rampant consolidation of healthcare conglomerates.

Not all practices are candidates for acquisition and affiliation with investor backed DPM companies. It is a matter of due course that a practice is thoroughly scrutinized before a purchase agreement is finalized. The 'under the hood' review of a practice can define its desirability. Financial performance of a practice is critical in determining valuation. Practices may be red flagged for accounting irregularities that are difficult to reconcile. Audits of billing and coding procedures may reveal policies that are inconsistent with prevailing rules and regulations, leaving the practice's true financial performance in doubt, and highlight the practice's risk for severe penalties from payer audits. A practice's policies and procedures and regulatory reporting may be antiquated or nonexistent. Evaluation of staff may reveal a hostile or toxic internal environment. Peer review by physicians is frequently integrated into the DPM's evaluation of potential acquisitions, and concerns expressed about a practice's quality of care and reputation can define the desirability for acquisition. Undoubtedly, there are private equity backed dermatology management companies where standards may vary. The level of intensity and attentiveness to external review is a good indicator of a DPMs commitment to high quality care.

The challenge of healthcare management is not unique to private practice. Academic dermatology also has been profoundly challenged by evolving administrative and regulatory demands. Support of the research, teaching and the clinical missions demand enhancing revenue. It is of no surprise that many of the same strategies taken by DPMs to enhance efficiencies and profitability are being deployed as academic dermatology undergoes a trend towards corporatization.[6]

## SUMMARY

Clearly this practice model has drawn significant attention within the specialty and by healthcare analysts. Such discourse is critical to any new model, and fervently held positions and in-depth analyses should receive close attention. However, key to any analysis is balance. Recent articles in the lay press may indict an investor role in healthcare. However, it is key also to understand that it is the individual DPM that requires thoughtful

analysis. It clearly is not a matter of "if you have seen one you've seen them all" but rather "if you've seen one, you've seen just one." Consolidation is a natural progression in any industry and that the best companies will survive and thrive, and that done well these DPMs can provide high quality care and value to all stakeholders, including providers, patients and investors.

Healthcare is an enormous segment of our economy, representing 18% of GDP. Profiting from this sector are providers, insurance companies, pharmaceutical and device manufacturers, health system executives, and many others. Enhanced profitability rewards the varied missions of stakeholders, be it the research and education mission of an academic medical center, the administrative leadership of a non-profit healthcare conglomerate, the shareholders of a for-profit enterprise, or the providers of a small group private practice. In the case of private equity companies, investment in consolidation of a fragmented specialty achieves enhanced profitability via deployment of management expertise, elimination of redundancy in overhead, and the leveraging of scale. In short, it is the strategies a company deploys to achieve profitability that warrant scrutiny. To be sure, safeguards for preserving the highest standards of medical practice can and should always be paramount, and in any affiliation agreement care should be taken to buttress these safeguards.

## REFERENCES

1. Konda S, Francis J, Grant-Kels JM. Future considerations for clinical dermatology in the setting of 21st century American reform: corporatization and the rise of private equity in dermatology. J Am Acad Dermatol 2019;81:287–96.
2. Resneck JS Jr. Dermatology practice consolidation fueled by private equity investment: potential consequences for the specialty and patients. JAMA Dermatol 2018;154:13–4.
3. Tan S, Seiger K, Renehan P, et al. Trends in private equity acquisition of dermatology practices in the United States. JAMA Dermatol 2019;155:1013–21.
4. Shanafelt TD. Physician well-being 2.0: Where are we and where are we going. Mayo Clin Proc 2021;96(10):2682–93.
5. Rosenstein AH. Understanding the psychology behind physician attitudes, behaviors, and engagement as the pathway to physician well-being. J Psychology and Clinical Psychiatry 2016;5:1–3.
6. DeWane ME, Mostow E, Grant-Kels JM. The corporatization of care in academic dermatology. Clin Dermatol 2020;38:289–95.
7. Braun RT, Bond AM, Qian Y. Private equity in dermatology: Effect on price, utilization, and spending. Health Aff 2021;40:1813–4.

# Private Equity
## The Bad and the Ugly

Sailesh Konda, MD*, Sagar Patel, MD, Joseph Francis, MD

## KEYWORDS

- Private equity • Corporate practice of medicine • Monopolistic practices
- Nonphysician practitioners • Cost of health care • Debt dependence
- Residency and fellowship programs • Professional and lifestyle considerations

## KEY POINTS

- Despite failures of private equity (PE) in the 1990s, dermatology PE-backed groups (DPEGs) have rapidly expanded over the last decade. Practice acquisitions are now declining, and mergers are on the rise.
- High interest rates can put pressure on the financial health of DPEGs.
- The US Federal Trade Commission and US Department of Justice may apply more regulatory scrutiny in coming years.
- DPEGs' primary focus on profits can lead to increased health care costs by overleveraging nonphysician practitioners and aggressive billing practices.
- Physician autonomy is diminished by DPEGs, which can increase physician burnout.

## INTRODUCTION

Private equity (PE) firms execute leveraged buyouts by acquiring target companies with a small amount of their own capital and a large amount of outside debt financing. They have steep "two and twenty" fees, which means they take up to 2% of the assets under management and 20% of profits above a predetermined threshold, known as the "hurdle rate." PE first became mainstream during the leveraged buyout boom in the 1980s, which subsequently busted in the early 1990s. Since the 1990s, PE has had multiple boom-and-bust periods that largely coincided with interest rates and the economic cycle. Herein, PE buyouts in dermatology will be discussed, including their effects on patients and physicians, and obstacles to their continued involvement.

## A FAILED EXPERIMENT AND ITS RESURRECTION

Physician practice management companies (PPMCs), many backed with PE investments,

started in the 1990s with billions of dollars of capital, promising synergy in larger groups, sophisticated clinical information systems to increase efficiency, and market power to counteract insurance companies.[1] The PPMC industry grew to over 30 publicly traded companies with a market capitalization more than $11 billion at its peak in January 1998.[2] However, PPMCs imploded soon thereafter.[1] Many groups filed for bankruptcy during the early 2000s, because they were overleveraged from rapid acquisitions and failed to achieve profitability from economies of scale.[2,3] In the aftermath, financial analysts concluded that the PPMCs are an impractical business model, add another layer of administrative costs into the health care system, and were similar to Ponzi and pyramid schemes.[1]

The recent PE boom was largely supported by dry powder, or committed capital awaiting investment, and low interest rates. This provided PE firms with cheap debt financing and profitable arbitrage opportunities across many industries. PE reentered medicine in the 2010s with a

Department of Dermatology, University of Florida College of Medicine, 4037 Northwest 86th Terrace, 4th Floor, Gainesville, FL 32606, USA
* Corresponding author.
E-mail address: sailesh.konda@dermatology.med.ufl.edu

Dermatol Clin 41 (2023) 597–610
https://doi.org/10.1016/j.det.2023.04.004
0733-8635/23/© 2023 Elsevier Inc. All rights reserved.

renewed focus on specialty-specific consolidation and the promise of value-based care. PE formed management service organizations (MSOs) to navigate around corporate practice of medicine (CPOM) laws and invested in many specialties, including dermatology.

Historically, since the early 2010s, there have been at least 40 dermatology PE-backed groups (DPEGs). Many dermatologists sold their practices to DPEGs for millions of dollars, are financially aligned with DPEGs, and serve as PE spokespeople for the promise of future equity returns.[4] Therefore, DPEGs pay a premium for the practices of influential leaders and social media influencers with the hope that they will use their positions to promote the DPEG. This may mislead younger dermatologists who are unaware of their respected mentors' allegiance. Past and current presidents and board members of the American Academy of Dermatology (AAD), American Society of Dermatologic Surgery, American College of Mohs Surgery, and even Dr. Pimple Popper have sold, work for, or have agreements with DPEGs.[5,6] The AAD updated its administrative regulations in 2019 to require disclosures of financial interests with PE.[7–9]

Some DPEG marketing materials tout that their physicians have held leadership offices in national and state medical associations and include words, such as "culture of quality," "the right fit," "freedom with stability," "physician-led," "trust," "true partnership," "practice sustainability," "physician autonomy," "loyalty to staff," and "peace of mind."[10,11] However, these marketing buzzwords were created by PE, not dermatologists. For example, a "true partnership" is not possible when one is an employee of a DPEG. As Cockrell and Dine of McGuireWoods LLP eloquently state, "In the PE cycle, one critical strategy that PE investors deliberate is the timing of the 'window of opportunity' so as to successfully exit an investment at the best possible purchase price, without being the last one standing."[12] Thus, DPEG marketing claims seem to be directly contrary to their main motivation.

## CIRCUMVENTING THE CORPORATE PRACTICE OF MEDICINE

The CPOM doctrine "prohibits corporations from practicing medicine or employing a physician to provide professional medical services." The CPOM doctrine was created because of obvious conflicts between corporate profits and patient interests.[13] Over 30 states have enacted laws prohibiting or restricting CPOM. PE has worked around this by investing in the medical service organization (MSO) and professional medical corporation (PMC) model to circumvent CPOM laws and structure relationships with physicians. PE invests in the MSO, which provides administrative and management support in exchange for a fixed fee or a percentage of medical practice revenue, and the PMC employs the physicians and NPPs.[4] The MSO should not interfere with the PMC, the practice of medicine, or a physician's medical judgment; however, CPOM is not strictly enforced and there are many anecdotes of this line being crossed in dermatology.[14–16]

Other specialties, specifically emergency medicine, are beginning to push back against PE using CPOM laws. Court filings in multiple states have called out emergency room PE-backed groups for "using doctor groups as straw men to sidestep CPOM laws."[17] Additionally, the American Academy of Emergency Medicine filed suit in federal court in California against Envision Healthcare Corporation to "prevent Envision from using captive medical groups, restrictive covenants in physician contracts, payment of consideration to acquire ED contracts, control over staffing, billing and payor contracts and similar practices which violate California's CPOM prohibition as well as other laws."[18] The trial is scheduled to commence in January 2024. It is supported by the California Medical Association, and its outcome could have national impact.

## MATURATION OF THE MARKET

DPEGs have increased their share of the dermatology market over the last decade as the physician arms race reaches new levels.[19] As they race to expand, DPEGs may even acquire nondermatologist physicians and close underperforming offices.[4,20,21] Most DPEGs have sold to other PE firms. A few have already failed and are no longer in existence, such as US Dermatology Medical Management, DermOne Dermatology, Select Dermatology, and TruDerm.[22] Failure is hugely disruptive to all concerned but, in particular, physicians may lose their share of accounts receivable and be eliminated from payrolls without recompense. It is difficult to get disenfranchised dermatologists to discuss such fiascos, as they are uniformly restricted by gag clauses.

Individual DPEGs usually claim that they are different from the rest. A familiar mantra is "when you have seen one DPEG you have seen one DPEG." However, they are all in different stages of evolution and become similar as they sell or flip, and the market demands conformity.[4] Because DPEGs have consolidated many of their geographic markets, the number of available practices to roll up has decreased. Deal activity has declined since 2020, and they are now entering an era of mergers to maintain continued transactions and investor returns.[23,24] For example, recent mergers include Skin and Beauty Center with DermCare Management, Water's Edge with Riverchase Dermatology (now rebranded as AQUA Dermatology), and West Dermatology with Platinum Dermatology Partners.[25-27] Some DPEGs will continue to merge to expand their geographic reach, and the next buyer may be another PE firm, a health care conglomerate, the public via an initial public offering, or an insurance company.[28]

These larger transactions are already becoming the norm, with Amazon, CVS, and Walgreens making multi-billion-dollar health care acquisitions.[29-33] Although benefits of vertical integration are often touted to obtain regulatory approval for these deals, there is significant concern regarding competition and the impact on patients when insurance, pharmacies, and clinics are all financially backed by a single entity, creating conflicts of interest.[34]

## MONOPOLISTIC PRACTICES

In October 2021, the University of Southern California-Brookings Schaeffer Initiative for Health Policy published a white paper that recommended enhanced enforcement under antitrust and employment laws to address consolidation and anticompetitive contracting practices imposed on acquired physicians.[35] In addition, a cross-sectional study examined geographic variations in PE and found that the Northeast, Florida, and Arizona had the highest PE penetration. Notably, PE penetration was highest in dermatology.[36]

Accordingly, the US Federal Trade Commission (FTC) and US Department of Justice (DOJ) are increasing their scrutiny of PE acquisitions in health care. Lina Khan, the Chair of the FTC has vowed a "muscular" antitrust approach to PE health care deals.[37] Similarly, Jonathan Kanter, head of DOJ's antitrust unit, noted PE firms that "hollow out or roll up an industry and essentially cash out" are "very much at odds with the law" and "the competition we're trying to protect."[38] The FTC and DOJ are increasing enforcement with a multipronged approach, which includes the following:

1. July 2020: The Hart-Scott-Rodino Antitrust Improvement Act (HSR Act) requires PE to notify the FTC and DOJ prior to transactions more than $94 million. However, PE firms typically acquire smaller, so-called "platform" practices, followed by add-on acquisitions, which are not subject to HSR reporting, and can "quietly increase market power and reduce competition."[39] Rohit Chopra, the previous Commissioner of the FTC, acknowledged these reporting deficiencies and need for increased monitoring.[39]

2. January 2021: The FTC has issued orders to 6 health insurance companies to provide information to retrospectively study physician practice consolidation from 2015 through 2020 and its effects on competition.[40]

3. January 2022: FTC-DOJ launched joint public inquiry soliciting input on modernizing merger guidelines to better detect and prevent anticompetitive deals, and comments were dominated by doctor's worries over PE deals and their negative impact. Many dermatologists complained about PE-backed consolidation, CPOM, and detrimental effects on patient care.[41-43] New guidelines are expected to be released in early 2023.

4. April 2022: The FTC-DOJ held a listening forum on the firsthand effects of mergers and acquisitions in health care, during which dermatology was discussed.[44]

5. June and October 2022: The FTC took action to protect competition in the veterinary industry and unanimously approved 2 separate orders against JAB Consumer Partners requiring divesture of clinics in multiple metropolitan areas. Furthermore, the FTC mandated strict prior approval and notice requirements for future acquisitions.[45,46]

6. October 2022: FTC began investigating PE-backed US Anesthesia Partners over whether it amassed too much power in some regional markets.[47]

7. October 2022: The DOJ enforced Section 2 of the Sherman Act for the first time in decades when a construction company contractor attempted to monopolize the market by proposing a "strategic partnership" with a competitor by allocating regional markets among themselves.[48,49] A potential parallel in the dermatology market is the Dermatology Practice Support Alliance (DPSA), a coalition of the largest DPEGs. When a DPSA member, DermOne Dermatology, dissolved in 2018, other DPSA members acquired DermOne Dermatology offices in New Jersey and Virginia and the medical records of Texas patients. Additionally, Schweiger Dermatology Group acquired The Dermatology Group in 2021, and both are DPSA members.[50]

8. January 2023: FTC proposed a rule to ban non-compete clauses, which hurt workers and harm

competition. The proposed rule would require employers to rescind existing noncompete clauses and actively inform workers that they are no longer in effect.[51,52] This would affect all practice models, including DPEGs, which depend on noncompete clauses in the contracts of employed dermatologists to keep physicians aligned and protect their financial relationships with patients. These noncompete clauses include the offices they work at or all the offices in a particular region or state.[4] PPMCs recognize they may be significantly impacted if the proposed rule is adopted and are planning on submitting comments to the FTC.[53] The US Chamber of Commerce, which represents some 3 million businesses, is prepared to sue if the FTC acts on its proposal.[54]

Given increased scrutiny in the current regulatory environment, it is unlikely that the tactics of DPEGS will remain under the radar.

## OVERLEVERAGING OF NONPHYSICIAN PRACTITIONERS

Research has shown that DPEGs employ a greater number of NPPs, have a higher ratio of NPPs to physicians compared with independently owned practices, and have significant yearly increases in the number of NPPs but not physicians after acquiring practices.[55–57] DPEGs also preferentially schedule new patient appointments with NPPs compared with non-PE owned practices and may misrepresent the qualifications of NPPs when patients are booking appointments.[58,59]

DPEGs may utilize NPPs because they cost less and perform more skin biopsies.[60–62] A flawed retrospective cohort study conducted by Advanced Dermatology and Cosmetic Surgery (ADCS) concluded that their in-house biopsy rates associated with nonpathologic cutaneous disease were not increasing; however, they included actinic keratoses as pathological cutaneous disease, implying they should be routinely biopsied, and excluded their entire NPP workforce from the analysis.[63]

DPEGs routinely expect employed dermatologists to supervise NPPs to the maximum extent allowable by state law with varying degrees of actual supervision. Dermatologists typically only receive a small percentage of the NPP's collections, with most going to the DPEG. Overall, dermatologic procedures billed independently by NPPs has significantly increased.[64] Some DPEGs also bill dermatologic services provided by NPPs under a physicians' National Provider Identifiers with incident-to billing. This maximizes revenue by increasing reimbursement for NPP services from 85% to 100% of the fee schedule and masks billing and utilization patterns of their NPPs. Dermatologists should be aware of the strict requirements for incident-to billing.[65]

## COST OF HEALTH CARE

Jack Resneck, a dermatologist who is the current AMA President, has expressed concerns about PE's effects on the specialty, profession, and patients, which could be irreversible.[34] Every DPEG relies heavily on utilization of lucrative CPT (current procedural terminology) codes. These include biopsies, pathology (including special stains), excisions, destructions, and Mohs surgery.[66] If one starts the process with NPPs (who perform more biopsies than physicians),[60–62] and are paid significantly less in salary, things become even more lucrative.

### Acquisition of Outliers

Konda and colleagues examined 2015 Medicare Part B physician payment data and found that some PE firms were acquiring outlier physicians performing extremely high mean numbers of skin biopsies per patient and were not performing due diligence when consolidating practices.[5] Additionally, the New York Times discovered that ADCS-owned Bedside Dermatology was employing NPPs in Michigan who were independently billing highly questionable intralesional injections on vulnerable nursing home patients, 75% of whom had dementia.[5,67]

### Postacquisition Changes

DPEGs evaluate prospective practice acquisitions during the due diligence phase with questionnaires that focus on financial metrics, to determine valuations and to see how to improve profit margins.[4] Braun and colleagues conducted a differences-in-differences study and analyzed commercial claims from 2012 to 2017. They found that PE consolidation leads to a modest 3% to 5% increase in the negotiated fee with insurers for routine visits.[57] The authors also concluded that DPEGs had no significant impact on total spending, overall use of dermatology procedures per patient, or specific high-volume and profitable procedures.[57] However, this conclusion was presumptive given several study limitations, and 2017, an active year for PE acquisitions, was not included in the data set.[68] In addition, their research was funded by the Physicians Foundation, which helps physicians navigate the changing health care system and has an adversarial stance toward insurers.[69]

Singh and colleagues conducted another differences-in-differences study, funded by the US National Institutes of Health. They examined dermatology, gastroenterology, and ophthalmology practices acquired by PE between 2016 and 2020.[70] An analysis of commercial insurance claims found PE-acquired practices had a 11% increase in negotiated fees and a 9.4% increase in the share of office visits for established patients that were billed as longer than 30 minutes face-to-face time. Dermatology-specific analyses found that, after PE acquisition, negotiated fees did not increase, share of established patients with higher-intensity visits increased, and evaluation and management and pathology service volume and total spending increased.[70] The authors postulate that this could be due to managerial changes or upcoding to optimize revenues. Their study did include 2017 in their data set but also has some limitations.

As demonstrated, DEPGs only have a modest or no increase in insurance payments after acquisition, which makes taking a 20% cut of profits almost entirely reliant on back office improvements. This seems unlikely.[71]

### Self-Referrals

The in-office ancillary services exemption of the Stark law allows practices to refer to themselves, which may encourage overutilization to generate more revenue. In a separate study, Singh used a discrete choice model and found that PE acquisitions of multispecialty physician practices increased self-referrals by 7%. These self-referrals seem to be driven by PE's managerial strategies.[72] These new referral patterns may be less responsive to patient needs or preferences and usually prevent competing specialists from accessing patient referrals[72] In fact, there have been multiple reports of DPEGs pressuring competing Mohs surgeons to sell their practices after DPEGs acquired and redirected their local referral sources.[66]

### The Glorification of Profits: Salve Lucrum

PE investments in hospitals, nursing homes, and anesthesia practice management companies have also been associated with increased health care costs.[73–77] Data such as these have created concern regarding quality of care and raise serious questions regarding how PE's fiduciary duty to their investors may compromise patient care.[78] US health care spending grew 2.7% to $4.3 trillion in 2021, accounting for 18.3% of gross domestic product, of which upwards of 30% can be attributed to administrative costs.[79–81] The quest for health care cost containment is incompatible with PE's goal of short-term profits.[82] Even American's Health Insurance Plans, a trade group for insurance companies, has released a report documenting specific concerns about PE investment in fee-for-service dermatology.[83] As stated in a recent viewpoint, the glorification of profit, salve lucrum, can have harmful effects on the health care system.[16,84]

### DEPENDENCE ON DEBT

A low interest rate environment favors PE, because investors can make sizable acquisitions and easily pay interest on the debt with revenue generated from acquired practices.[85,86] DPEGs can quickly acquire practices, patch them together, and sell to the next highest bidder at inflated valuations. As recently as February 2022, Forefront Dermatology was acquired by Partners Group, a Swiss-based PE firm, at a valuation of $1.5 billion.[87] Since March 2022, interest rates have been quickly increasing, which can be expected to put a damper on PE acquisitions.[88–91]

Most of PE debt holdings are priced at a variable rate, which means when rates go higher, DPEGs spend more of their revenue servicing debt.[92] This has limited exit opportunities and created investment illiquidity, which can affect physicians with equity stakes in DPEGs. When PE purchases a practice, much of the purchase price paid to the physicians is equity in the new corporation with the promise of major profits when the conglomerate is sold in a few years. It has become more common to require physicians to retain up to 100% of their equity stake rather than cash out during a subsequent sale or merger. delaying their promised second bite of the apple.[93] This can limit the options of employed dermatologists, as they may have to forfeit equity if they leave the DPEG.[34,93]

DPEG debt valuations can fluctuate depending on the market's opinion of ability to repay debt obligations. Memon and colleagues conducted a cross-sectional study of public financial statements from August 2016 to August 2021. Even during an era of low interest rates, a significant decrease in debt valuations of DPEGs before and during the pandemic was found.[22] For example, using debt valuations, US Dermatology Partners' (USDP) failure to repay a $377 million direct lender loan in January 2020 could be predicted, as they had the most heavily discounted debt of examined DPEGs.[22,94] However, USDP and other DPEGs still want to be small businesses when it suits them; they took over $26 million in forgivable Small Business Administration Paycheck Protection

Program loans in 2020.[22] Rapid rate increases may put further pressure on DPEGs to prioritize servicing debt over expansion during a period of Medicare cuts.[95] Debt valuations of some DPEGs can be calculated by reviewing annual and quarterly reports filed with the US Securities and Exchange Commission; this should be investigated prior to signing on or selling.

## TRAINING UNDER PRIVATE EQUITY

The health care industry increasingly values Accreditation Council for Graduate Medical Education-accredited residency and fellowship programs as an asset.[96] DPEGs highly value practices with associated training programs, which can serve as pipelines for their future workforce.[5,97] Some DPEGs have even structured resident salaries as partial loans, and, upon completion of training, trainees have the option of paying these loans back in their entirety or signing employment contracts with restrictive covenants.[5] PE has steadily acquired hospitals and practices associated with training programs. Disturbingly, Rush University Medical Center has agreed to have clinical and academic affiliations with a DPEG in exchange for a minority stake in the DPEG.[98] While this trend has gone largely unnoticed, the US Centers for Medicare and Medicaid Services (CMS) consider the auction and sale of CMS-funded residents and fellows illegal. In the case of Hahnemann University Hospital, CMS appealed the $55 million sale of Hahnemann's residency program to a coalition of health systems led by Thomas Jefferson University.[99,100]

Additionally, the American Medical Association adopted a resolution in November 2022 to address PE's growing impact on residency training. The resolution encourages GME programs and institutions to be transparent on mergers and closures relating to PE acquisitions, and this information should be made available to current and prospective trainees.[101,102] The AMA also encourages public statements from physician societies about PE's impact on residency training to heighten awareness.[101] In dermatology, there has already been a closure of a DPEG associated with a residency program.[5,103] **Table 1** lists known training programs associated with DPEGs.

## PROFESSIONAL AND LIFESTYLE CONSIDERATIONS

Physician burnout is on the rise and is becoming more common in today's environment.[104] Although some may attribute this to generational differences, the authors believe there are several other more relevant considerations. Physicians have dedicated almost a decade beyond college to training; a meaningful employment arrangement can have a huge impact on happiness.

The origin of burnout (**Fig. 1**) begins when students seeking to pursue careers in the health professions are put into debt by the ever-increasing number of expensive for-profit colleges and medical schools.[105] In a Medscape survey, half of resident respondents owed more than $200,000 in medical school loans, with 26% owing more than $300,000.[106] After completing their training, students usually only have a few months before the first loan payments are due. The offer of a high base salary may appear to be a lifeline. Residents typically do not have the money to afford a legal review of their contract or time and leverage to negotiate. Many residents believe they will only work there for a few years until they pay off their loans but become invested in the community (eg, spouse, house, and children). Later, they realize all the compromises that accompany a high base salary. Additionally, DPEG contracts are notoriously restrictive and punitive, making leaving their employment difficult.

In his book Outliers, author Malcolm Gladwell discusses the 3 components needed to make work meaningful and presumably, less likely to lead to burnout.[107] These are: autonomy, challenge, and a direct link between the way one is paid and the amount of effort one puts in. PE diminishes all three.

### Autonomy

1. DPEGs decrease one's autonomy by controlling patient volume and how much time one gets to see a patient. They can typically require their physician employees to practice in several offices and even fly to multiple states. DPEGs can specify, or strongly suggest, which pharmacy and referring doctors their employees should use.
2. One may not be able to control the level of staffing in the office. To cut costs, DPEGs have been known to cut administrative staff and benefits. Benefits may change with each sale or merger of the conglomerate.
3. One may not be given a choice as to whether one will supervise NPPs and for how many one is responsible.

### Effort/Reward and Challenge

PE may remove the direct link between effort and reward by paying one a fixed salary no matter how much one works, which they also control. Sometimes this is paired with unobtainable bonus targets. Compensation terms can also change

**Table 1**
Accreditation Council for Graduate Medical Education-accredited residency and fellowship programs associated with dermatology private equity-backed groups

| Program[a] | Location | Residency/Fellowship[2] | Associated DPEG(s) |
|---|---|---|---|
| Kansas City University GME Consortium (KCU-GME Consortium)/ADCS-Orlando Program | Maitland, Florida | D | Advanced Dermatology and Cosmetic Surgery |
| Larkin Community Hospital Program | South Miami, Florida | D, MSDO | DermCare Management; Skin and Cancer Associates and the Center for Cosmetic Enhancement; MedSpa Partners |
| Larkin Community Hospital Palm Springs Campus Program | Hialeah, Florida | D, MSDO, DP | DermCare Management; Skin and Cancer Associates and the Center for Cosmetic Enhancement; MedSpa Partners |
| Beaumont Health (Trenton) Program | Trenton, Michigan | D | Advanced Dermatology and Cosmetic Surgery |
| Hackensack University Medical Center (Palisades) Program | North Bergen, New Jersey | D | Schweiger Dermatology Group |
| St John's Episcopal Hospital-South Shore Program | Far Rockaway, New York | D | The Dermatology Specialists |
| St. Barnabas Hospital | Bronx, New York | D | The Dermatology Specialists |
| OhioHealth/Riverside Methodist Hospital Program | Columbus, Ohio | D | Dermatologists of Central States; QualDerm Partners |
| Wright State University School of Medicine | Fairborn, Ohio | D | Dermatologists of Central States |
| Samaritan Health Services - Corvallis Program | Salem, Oregon | D, MSDO | Frontier Derm Partners |
| Surgical Dermatology Group Program | Vestavia Hills, Alabama | MSDO | AQUA Dermatology |
| Laser & Skin Surgery Center of New York | New York, New York | MSDO | NavaDerm Partners |
| Zitelli and Brodland Clinic Program | Pittsburgh, Pennsylvania | MSDO | QualDerm Partners |

*Abbreviations:* D, dermatology residency; DP, dermatopathology fellowship; MSDO, micrographic surgery and dermatologic oncology fellowship.
[a] Programs were included if any time was spent training at a DPEG site.

whenever they want them to–as witnessed during the pandemic. The value of any effort one puts into building the practice with hopes of becoming a partner is also gone when PE purchases the practice while one is an employed physician.

The challenges of working with diverse patient population can also be curtailed by PE. Some of these groups limit the acceptance of insurance plans that cater to the poor.[108] This inequity is also counter to the DPEGs claims of improving access.

Complex medical dermatology and challenging surgical cases may be referred out to other specialists or universities to maximize patient flow.

All these factors considered, it is not surprising that research has found that there is a higher probability of physicians entering and exiting DPEGs than independent practices. These findings suggest a higher degree of workforce turnover, which may be due to dissatisfaction.[56] When there is turnover, a physician is more likely to be replaced by an

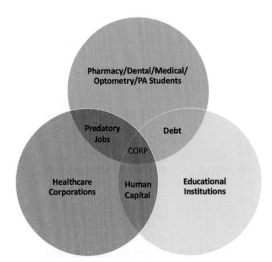

**Fig. 1.** Corporatization of health care (*center*) originating from the interplay between students, educational institutions, and health care corporations.

NPP at a DPEG.[56] Also remember that with the grow and flip model, DPEGs cannot survive without constant infusions of young dermatologists to see the patients while their older dermatologists scale back. Dermatologists in DPEGs also see higher volumes of patients[57,70] compared with independent practices. All together, these factors may also contribute to physician burnout.

### Other Factors Contributing to Burnout

As this younger generation values lifestyle considerations over monetary compensation, the high replacement ratios of young physicians and NPPs found by Zhu and colleagues may also indicate that the incentives offered by DPEGs cannot counter the negatives of working for them. The increased use of NPPs by PE may not be caused by a shortage of physicians but merely a shortage of physicians who want to work for them. Most surveyed residents are wary of working for DPEGs and believe PE strongly worsens physician autonomy, quality of patient care, and long-term salary.[109] Even physician recruiters understand this and now advertise job postings as "not private equity." DPEGs aggressively enforce nondisparagement and nondisclosure agreements and attempt to quell skepticism and negative media attention.[23] They perpetually rebrand themselves to hide their past, which allows them to maintain a better public image that they use for recruiting. If one does have a falling out with them, paying attorneys to ensure one's silence is much more effective for them than marketing dollars.[16]

DPEG physician contracts are typically intricate and often poisonous with extraordinary noncompete clauses and financial punishments. These contracts are typically reassignable, giving the current group consent to sell one's services to the next owner. The noncompete clause, one's personal debt, links to the community, lack of legal and administrative know-how, and time-based financial incentives keep one from jumping ship before the flip. In fact, one risks being sold to PE with any private practice one enters as an employed physician; there has been a rise of regional private mega-practices that intend to sell to PE. The new reality is that these intentions may not be communicated, and one may not know who one's employer will be every few years. Any physician contemplating employment by a DPEG must have his or her contract reviewed by an attorney who specializes in medical contracts. DPEGs will negotiate much more readily when one is represented by an attorney.

### SUMMARY

In his recent book, The Myth of Private Equity, Jeffrey Hooke, a former PE executive and critic, explains how PE is "self-mythologizing" with a "penchant for secrecy."[110] Although DPEGs have claimed consolidation will lead to more cost-efficient health care through economies of scale, higher quality health care, and improved health care delivery, these theoretical benefits have not been demonstrated in practice.[111] Claims of efficiency and improved outcomes are not supported by data, which show that these efficiencies generally never materialize, quality of care often worsens, and health care costs increase.[70,111]

The decade of low interest rates has ended; the music has stopped, and the free money party has come to an end. The International PE Market community met in Cannes in January 2023 under the theme "Reality Check," and the consensus was that 2023 will be the year that valuations fall back down to earth.[112–114] Future PE acquisitions may decrease with higher interest rates and scrutiny from the FTC. If allowed to grow unchecked, DPEGs may end up selling dermatologists to the very entities they sought to counteract, health care conglomerates, insurance companies, and universities.[98]

Interest in, training, and recruitment of young dermatologists are critical to sustaining the DPEG business model, which is why some heavily market to this demographic with social media influencers.[115] One of DPEGs' main talking points to young physicians is that there is strength in large organizations and that they have special relationships with insurers to make sure one gets paid more, but as discussed earlier, this is rarely the case. Behind the smoke and mirrors, it really is all about money, control of the specialty, and an exit strategy for older physicians.[116]

PE offers itself as salvation for declining reimbursements while at the same time driving overutilization.[71] Remember this the next time they make an offer not to be refused. Dermatologists seeking a meaningful career and avoidance of burnout should be aware of the current challenges in today's job market and the deceptive allure of working for PE. Making uninformed choices early on can result in years of unhappiness and missed opportunities.

## FUNDING SOURCES

There are no funding sources for this work.

## CONFLICTS OF INTEREST

The authors have no conflict of interest to declare.

## REFERENCES

1. Reinhardt UE. The rise and fall of the physician practice management industry. Health Aff 2000;19:42–55.
2. Luria N, Hagood G. Industry voices - private equity may be repeating mistakes with physician practice management companies. Available at: https://www.fiercehealthcare.com/practices/industry-voices-private-equity-may-be-repeating-mistakes-physician-practice-management. Accessed January 25, 2023.
3. Lowes R. Physician practice management companies. Going.going. Available at: https://www.medicaleconomics.com/view/physician-practice-management-companies-goinggoing. Accessed January 25, 2023.
4. Konda S, Francis J. The evolution of private equity in dermatology. Clin Dermatol 2020;38:275–83.
5. Konda S, Francis J, Motaparthi K, et al. Group for Research of Corporatization and Private Equity in Dermatology. Future considerations for clinical dermatology in the setting of 21st century American policy reform: corporatization and the rise of private equity in dermatology. J Am Acad Dermatol 2019;81:287–96.e8.
6. Cross Keys Capital advises Dr. Pimple Popper and Skin Physicians & Surgeons in their partnership with Forefront Dermatology. Available at: https://www.globenewswire.com/en/news-release/2021/12/16/2353712/0/en/Cross-Keys-Capital-Advises-Dr-Pimple-Popper-and-Skin-Physicians-Surgeons-in-Their-Partnership-with-Forefront-Dermatology.html. Accessed January 25, 2023.
7. Waldman R, Kelsey A, Grant-Kels JM. Comment on: "Conflicts of interest for physician owners of private equity-owned medical practices". J Am Acad Dermatol 2020;82:e33.
8. AAD COI disclosures and private equity resolution. Available at: https://www.change.org/p/american-academy-of-dermatology-aad-private-equity-resolution. Accessed January 25, 2023.
9. American Academy of Dermatology Association. Administrative regulations: disclosure of outside interests and management of conflicts of interest. Available at: https://server.aad.org//Forms/Policies/Uploads/AR/AR%20-%20Disclosure%20of%20Outside%20Interests%20and%20Management%20of%20Conflicts%20of%20Interest.pdf. Accessed January 25, 2023.
10. QualDerm Partners. Available at: https://www.qualderm.com/. Accessed January 25, 2023.
11. QualDerm Partners. By the numbers. Available at: https://www.qualderm.com/wp-content/uploads/2022/09/QDP-By-the-Numbers-09.30.22.pdf. Accessed January 25, 2023.
12. Cockrell GC, Dine EE. Private equity investment in dermatology practices: adding more "skin to the game" through a cosmetic service line. Health Care Law Mon 2019;2019(4):2–7.
13. American Medical Association. Issue brief: corporate practice of medicine. Available at: https://www.ama-assn.org/sites/default/files/media-browser/premium/arc/corporate-practice-of-medicine-issue-brief_1.pdf. Accessed January 14, 2018.
14. Francis J, Konda S, Lain E. Private equity and venture capital-backed practice models. In: Dover JS, Mariwalla K, editors. The business of dermatology. 1st edition. New York: Thieme; 2020. p. 82–96.
15. Perlberg H. How private equity is ruining American health care. Available at: https://www.bloomberg.com/news/features/2020-05-20/private-equity-is-ruining-health-care-covid-is-making-it-worse. Accessed January 25, 2023.
16. Morgenson G. 'Get that money!' Dermatologist says patient care suffered after private equity-backed firm bought her practice. Available at: https://www.nbcnews.com/health/health-care/get-money-dermatologist-says-patient-care-suffered-private-equity-back-rcna9152. Accessed January 25, 2023.
17. Wolfson BJ. ED doctors call private equity staffing practices illegal and seek to ban them. Available at: https://www.medscape.com/viewarticle/986274. Accessed January 25, 2023.
18. American Academy of Emergency Medicine. AAEM-PG files suit against Envision Healthcare alleging the illegal Corporate Practice of Medicine. Available at: https://www.aaem.org/current-news/aaem-pg-files-suit-against-envision-healthcare-alleging-the-illegal-corporate-practice-of-medicine. Accessed January 25, 2023.
19. Tan S, Seiger K, Renehan P, et al. Trends in private equity acquisition of dermatology practices in the United States. JAMA Dermatol 2019;155:1013–21.
20. QualDerm Partners. QualDerm further expands its quality-driven network in North Carolina. Available at: https://www.qualderm.com/qualderm-further-expands-its-quality-driven-network-in-north-carolina-2/. Accessed January 25, 2023.

21. Advanced dermatology and cosmetic surgery. Brian Gelb, MD. Available at: https://www.advancedderm.com/about-us/our-providers/brian-gelb-md. Accessed January 25, 2023.

22. Memon R, Memon A, Francis J, et al. Trends in debt valuations of private equity-backed dermatology groups before and during the COVID-19 Pandemic. JAMA Dermatol 2022;158:395–403.

23. PitchBook. Established private equity healthcare provider plays. Available at: https://files.pitchbook.com/website/files/pdf/Established_Private_Equity_Healthcare_Provider_Plays.pdf. Accessed January 25, 2023.

24. PitchBook. Healthcare services report. Available at: https://files.pitchbook.com/website/files/pdf/Q4_2022_Healthcare_Services_Report.pdf. Accessed February 6, 2023.

25. Hildred Capital Management and Gemini Investors announce recapitalization of DermCare and Skin & Beauty Center. Available at: https://www.businesswire.com/news/home/20191010005761/en/Hildred-Capital-Management-and-Gemini-Investors-Announce-Recapitalization-of-DermCare-and-Skin-Beauty-Center. Accessed January 25, 2023.

26. Water's Edge Dermatology and Riverchase Dermatology rebrand as AQUA Dermatology. Available at: https://www.prnewswire.com/news-releases/waters-edge-dermatology-and-riverchase-dermatology-rebrand-as-aqua-dermatology-301517519.html. Accessed January 25, 2023.

27. Sun Capital Partners and Sterling Partners merge West Dermatology and Platinum Dermatology Partners. Available at: https://www.businesswire.com/news/home/20220621005369/en/Sun-Capital-Partners-and-Sterling-Partners-Merge-West-Dermatology-and-Platinum-Dermatology-Partners. Accessed January 25, 2023.

28. Mathews AW. Physicians, hospitals meet their new competitor: insurer-owned clinics. Available at: https://www.wsj.com/articles/physicians-hospitals-meet-their-new-competitor-insurer-owned-clinics-11582473600. Accessed January 25, 2023.

29. Landi H. Amazon scoops up primary care company One Medical in deal valued at $3.9B. Available at: https://www.fiercehealthcare.com/health-tech/amazon-shells-out-39b-primary-care-startup-one-medical. Accessed January 25, 2023.

30. Japsen B. CVS beats Amazon and rivals for Signify Health with winning $8 billion bid. Available at: https://www.forbes.com/sites/brucejapsen/2022/09/05/cvs-health-bests-amazon-rivals-for-signify-health-with-8-billion-bid. Accessed January 25, 2023.

31. Japsen B. Walgreens-backed VillageMD and Cigna's Evernorth to buy clinic operator Summit Health for nearly $9 billion. Available at: https://www.forbes.com/sites/brucejapsen/2022/11/07/walgreens-backed-villagemd-and-cignas-evernorth-to-buy-summit-health-for-nearly-9-billion. Accessed January 25, 2023.

32. Mathews AW. CVS reaches $10.6 billion deal to buy clinic owner Oak Street Health. Available at: https://www.wsj.com/articles/cvs-earnings-report-oak-street-health-merger-11675835625. Accessed February 10, 2023.

33. Mak T. One Medical employees say concierge care provider is putting profits over patients. Available at: https://www.npr.org/2021/08/04/1016561613/one-medical-employees-say-concierge-care-provider-is-putting-profits-over-patien. Accessed January 25, 2023.

34. Resneck JS. Dermatology Practice Consolidation Fueled by Private Equity Investment: Potential Consequences for the Specialty and Patients. JAMA Dermatol 2018;154:13–4.

35. Fuse Brown EC, Adler L, Duffy E, et al Private equity investment as a divining rod for market failure: policy responses to harmful physician practice acquisitions. Available at: https://www.brookings.edu/essay/private-equity-investment-as-a-divining-rod-for-market-failure-policy-responses-to-harmful-physician-practice-acquisitions/. Accessed January 25, 2023.

36. Singh Y, Zhu JM, Polsky D, et al. Geographic variation in private equity penetration across select office-based physician specialties in the US. JAMA Health Forum 2022;3:e220825.

37. Palma S, Vandevelde M, Fontanella-Khan J. Lina Khan vows 'muscular' US antitrust approach on private equity deals. Available at: https://www.ft.com/content/ef9e4ce8-ab9a-45b3-ad91-7877f0e1c797. Accessed January 25, 2023.

38. Palma S, Fontanella-Khan J. Crackdown on buyout deals coming, warns top US antitrust enforcer. Available at: https://www.ft.com/content/7f4cc882-1444-4ea3-8a31-c382364aace1. Accessed January 25, 2023.

39. Federal Trade Commission. Statement of Commissioner Rohit Chopra regarding private equity roll-ups and the Hart-Scott-Rodino Annual Report to Congress. Available at: https://www.ftc.gov/legal-library/browse/cases-proceedings/public-statements/statement-commissioner-rohit-chopra-regarding-private-equity-roll-ups-hart-scott-rodino-annual. Accessed January 25, 2023.

40. Federal Trade Commission. FTC to study the impact of physician group and healthcare facility mergers. Available at: https://www.ftc.gov/news-events/news/press-releases/2021/01/ftc-study-impact-physician-group-healthcare-facility-mergers. Accessed January 25, 2023.

41. Federal Trade Commission. Federal Trade Commission and Justice Department seek to strengthen

enforcement against illegal mergers. Available at: https://www.ftc.gov/news-events/news/press-releases/2022/01/federal-trade-commission-justice-department-seek-strengthen-enforcement-against-illegal-mergers. Accessed January 25, 2023.

42. Federal Trade Commission. Request for information on merger enforcement. Available at: https://www.regulations.gov/document/FTC-2022-0003-0001. Accessed January 25, 2023.

43. Koenig B. Doctors' worries over PE deals dominate merger comments. Available at: https://www.law360.com/articles/1476116/doctors-worries-over-pe-deals-dominate-merger-comments. Accessed January 25, 2023.

44. Federal Trade Commission. FTC-DOJ Listening Forum - Health Care- April 14, 2022. Available at: https://www.ftc.gov/media/ftc-doj-listening-forum-health-care-april-14-2022. Accessed January 25, 2023.

45. Federal Trade Commission. FTC acts to protect pet owners from private equity firm's anticompetitive acquisition of veterinary services clinics. Available at: https://www.ftc.gov/news-events/news/press-releases/2022/06/ftc-acts-protect-pet-owners-private-equity-firms-anticompetitive-acquisition-veterinary-services. Accessed January 25, 2023.

46. Federal Trade Commission. FTC approves final order against JAB Consumer Partners to protect pet owners from private equity firm's rollup of veterinary services clinics. Available at: https://www.ftc.gov/news-events/news/press-releases/2022/10/ftc-approves-final-order-against-jab-consumer-partners-protect-pet-owners-private-equity-firms. Accessed January 25, 2023.

47. Michaels D. FTC probes market power of one of country's biggest anesthesia providers. Available at: https://www.wsj.com/articles/ftc-probes-market-power-of-one-of-countrys-biggest-anesthesia-providers-11664644401. Accessed January 25, 2023.

48. Murphy JP, Lee AJ, Thompson PM. DOJ prosecutes attempted collusion among business competitors for the first time in decades. Available at: https://www.mwe.com/insights/doj-issues-first-criminal-prosecution-of-section-2-of-the-sherman-act-in-decades/. Accessed January 25, 2023.

49. Department of Justice. Executive pleads guilty to criminal attempted monopolization. Available at: https://www.justice.gov/opa/pr/executive-pleads-guilty-criminal-attempted-monopolization. Accessed January 25, 2023.

50. Schweiger Dermatology Group. Schweiger Dermatology Group expands footprint in New Jersey with acquisition of The Derm Group. Available at: https://www.schweigerderm.com/skin-care-articles/press-releases/schweiger-dermatology-group-expands-footprint-in-new-jersey-with-acquisition-of-the-derm-group/#. Accessed January 25, 2023.

51. Federal Trade Commission. FTC proposes rule to ban noncompete clauses, which hurt workers and harm competition. Available at: https://www.ftc.gov/news-events/news/press-releases/2023/01/ftc-proposes-rule-ban-noncompete-clauses-which-hurt-workers-harm-competition. Accessed January 25, 2023.

52. Michaels D. FTC proposes banning noncompete clauses for workers. Available at: https://www.wsj.com/articles/ftc-proposes-banning-noncompete-clauses-for-workers-11672900586. Accessed January 25, 2023.

53. McDermott Will & Emery. PPMs, take note: FTC proposed rule banning noncompetes may have significant industry impact. Available at: https://www.mwe.com/insights/ppms-take-note-ftc-proposed-rule-banning-noncompetes-may-have-significant-industry-impact/. Accessed January 25, 2023.

54. Cox C. US Chamber of Commerce threatens to sue the FTC over proposed ban on noncompete clauses. Available at: https://www.cnbc.com/2023/01/12/us-chamber-of-commerce-threatens-to-sue-the-ftc-over-proposed-ban-on-noncompete-clauses.html. Accessed January 25, 2023.

55. Skaljic M, Lipoff JB. Association of private equity ownership with increased employment of advanced practice professionals in outpatient dermatology offices. J Am Acad Dermatol 2021; 84:1178–80.

56. Bruch JD, Foot C, Singh Y, et al. Workforce composition in private equity-acquired versus non-private equity-acquired physician practices. Health Aff 2023;42:121–9.

57. Braun RT, Bond AM, Qian Y, et al. Private equity in dermatology: effect on price, utilization, and spending. Health Aff 2021;40:727–35.

58. Creadore A, Desai S, Li SJ, et al. Insurance acceptance, appointment wait time, and dermatologist access across practice types in the US. JAMA Dermatol 2021;157:181–8.

59. Creadore A, Desai S, Li SJ, et al. Prevalence of misrepresentation of nonphysician clinicians at dermatology clinics. Cureus 2021;13:e18793.

60. Nault A, Zhang C, Kim K, et al. Biopsy use in skin cancer diagnosis: comparing dermatology physicians and advanced practice professionals. JAMA Dermatol 2015;151:899–902.

61. Anderson AM, Matsumoto M, Saul MI, et al. Accuracy of skin cancer diagnosis by physician assistants compared with dermatologists in a large health care system. JAMA Dermatol 2018;18.

62. Privalle A, Havighurst T, Kim K, et al. Number of skin biopsies needed per malignancy: comparing the utilization of skin biopsies among dermatologists and non-dermatologist clinicians. J Am Acad Dermatol 2020;82(1):110–6.

63. Solomon JA, Oswalt M, Nodzenski M, et al. Assessing skin biopsy rates for histologic findings indicative of nonpathological cutaneous disease. Dermatol Surg 2019;45:640–9.

64. Qi Q, Hibler BP, Coldiron B, et al. Analysis of dermatologic procedures billed independently by non-physician practitioners in the United States. J Am Acad Dermatol 2023;88(5):e203–9.

65. Centers for Medicare and Medicaid Services. Medicare benefit policy manual. Chapter 15. Covered medical and other health services. Available at: https://www.cms.gov/Regulations-and-Guidance/Guidance/Manuals/downloads/bp102c15.pdf. Accessed January 25, 2023.

66. Lain E. 13.3.4 life after the sale. In: Dover JS, Mariwalla M, editors. The business of dermatology. 1st edition. New York, NY: Thieme; 2020. p. 95–6.

67. Hafner K, Palmer G. Skin cancers rise, along with questionable treatments. New York Times; 2017. Health. Available at: https://www.nytimes.com/2017/11/20/health/dermatology-skin-cancer.html. Accessed January 25, 2023.

68. Francis J, Konda S. Private equity in dermatology. Health Aff 2021;40:1813.

69. The Physicians Foundation. Our hisitory. Available at: https://physiciansfoundation.org/about/our-history/. Accessed January 25, 2023.

70. Singh Y, Song Z, Polsky D, et al. Association of private equity acquisition of physician practices with changes in health care spending and utilization. JAMA Health Forum 2022;3(9):e222886.

71. Beaulieu ND, Chernew ME, McWilliams JM, et al. Organization and performance of US health systems. JAMA 2023;329:325–35.

72. Singh Y. Can private equity buy referrals? Evidence from multispecialty physician practice acquisition. Available at: https://www.yashaswinisingh.com/files/PE_Referrals_Singh_JMP.pdf. Accessed January 25, 2023.

73. Braun RT, Jung H, Casalino LP, et al. Association of private equity investment in US nursing homes with the quality and cost of care for long-stay residents. JAMA Health Forum 2021;2:e213817.

74. Bruch JD, Gondi S, Song Z. Changes in hospital income, use, and quality associated with private equity acquisition. JAMA Intern Med 2020;180:1428–35.

75. La Forgia A, Bond AM, Braun RT, et al. Association of physician management companies and private equity investment with commercial health care prices paid to anesthesia practitioners. JAMA Intern Med 2022;182:396–404.

76. Gupta A, Howell ST, Yannelis C, et al. Does private equity investment in healthcare benefit patients? Evidence from nursing homes. Available at: https://www.nber.org/papers/w28474. Accessed January 25, 2023.

77. Appelbaum E, Batt R. Available at: https://cepr.net/report/private-equity-buyouts-in-healthcare-who-wins-who-loses/. Accessed January 25, 2023.

78. Himmelstein DU, Woolhandler S. Privatization in a publicly funded health care system: the US experience. Int J Health Serv 2008;38:407–19.

79. Centers for Medicare and Medicaid Services. Historical health expenditure 2021. Available at: https://www.cms.gov/research-statistics-data-and-systems/statistics-trends-and-reports/nationalhealth expenddata/nhe-fact-sheet. Accessed January 25, 2023.

80. Tollen L, Keating E, Weil A. How administrative spending contributes to excess US health spending. Available at: https://www.healthaffairs.org/do/10.1377/forefront.20200218.375060/. Accessed January 25, 2023.

81. Woolhandler S, Campbell T, Himmelstein DU. Costs of health care administration in the United States and Canada. N Engl J Med 2003;349:768–75.

82. Altman DE, Levitt L. The sad history of health care cost containment as told in one chart. Health Aff (Millwood) 2002;Suppl web exclusives:W83–4.

83. America's Health Insurance Plans. Private equity investment in fee-for-service health care: lower quality at higher costs. Available at: https://www.ahip.org/documents/202208-AHIP-Private-Equity-Issue-Brief_v04.pdf. Accessed January 25, 2023.

84. Berwick DM. Salve lucrum: the existential threat of greed in US health care. JAMA 2023;329(8):629–30.

85. Kaplan SN, Stromberg P. Leveraged buyouts and private equity. J Econ Perspect 2009;23:121–46.

86. Gottfried M. Buyout boom gains steam in record year for private equity. Available at: https://www.wsj.com/articles/buyout-boom-gains-steam-in-record-year-for-private-equity-11638095402. Accessed January 25, 2023.

87. Sovereign Wealth Fund Institute. OMERS PE sells Forefront Dermatology to Partners Group. Available at: https://www.swfinstitute.org/news/91289/omers-pe-sells-forefront-dermatology-to-partners-group. Accessed January 25, 2023.

88. Tepper T. Federal funds rate history 1990 to 2022. Available at: https://www.forbes.com/advisor/investing/fed-funds-rate-history/. Accessed January 25, 2023.

89. US Bureau of Labor Statistics. Consumer prices up 9.1 percent over the year ended June 2022, largest increase in 40 years. Available at: https://www.bls.gov/opub/ted/2022/consumer-prices-up-9-1-percent-over-the-year-ended-june-2022-largest-increase-in-40-years.htm. Accessed January 25, 2023.

90. Cooper L. Leveraged loans become pricey, robbing buyout boom of momentum. Available at: https://www.wsj.com/articles/leveraged-loans-become-pricey-robbing-buyout-boom-of-momentum-11654767000. Accessed January 25, 2023.

91. The Economist. Private equity may be heading for a fall. Available at: https://www.economist.com/business/2022/07/07/private-equity-may-be-heading-for-a-fall. Accessed January 25, 2023.

92. O'Brien B. For private equity firms, rising rates are a double-edged sword. Available at: https://www.thestreet.com/investing/stocks/rising-rates-a-double-edged-sword-for-private-equity-13595991. Accessed January 25, 2023.

93. Strode RD. Learnings from recent physician practice private equity transactions. Available at: https://www.foley.com/en/insights/publications/2022/12/physician-practice-private-equity-transactions. Accessed January 25, 2023.

94. Butler K, Perlberg H. US Dermatology defaults on $377 million direct lender loan. Available at: https://www.bloomberg.com/news/articles/2020-01-31/u-s-dermatology-defaults-on-377-million-direct-lender-loan. Accessed January 25, 2023.

95. Lubell J. Medicare physician pay system needs a real fix—not more patches. Available at: https://www.ama-assn.org/practice-management/medicare-medicaid/medicare-physician-pay-system-needs-real-fix-not-more-patches. Accessed January 25, 2023.

96. Kadakia KT, Zheng J, Bruch JD, et al. Comparison of the financial and operational characteristics of for-profit and nonprofit hospitals receiving federal graduate medical education payments, 2011-2020. JAMA 2023;329:173–5.

97. The Healthcare MSO Conference. Private equity investment objectives & structuring MSOs for an exit. Available at: https://www.youtube.com/watch?v=AxPDB_TbVCI. Accessed January 25, 2023.

98. Finnegan J. Multistate dermatology practice affiliates with Rush University Medical Center. Available at: https://www.fiercehealthcare.com/practices/multi-state-dermatology-practice-affiliates-rush-university-medical-center. Accessed January 25, 2023.

99. Brubaker H. Hahnemann residency program sale approved by bankruptcy judge in controversial decision. Available at: https://www.inquirer.com/business/health/hahnemann-bankruptcy-residency-sale-judge-approves-cms-20190905.html. Accessed January 25, 2023.

100. George J. Feds appeal $55M sale of Hahnemann's residency program. Available at: https://www.bizjournals.com/philadelphia/news/2019/09/12/federal-government-appeals-approval-of-55m-sale-of.html. Accessed March 7, 2023.

101. Murphy B. Address private equity's growing impact on residency training. Available at: https://www.ama-assn.org/education/gme-funding/address-private-equity-s-growing-impact-residency-training. Accessed January 25, 2023.

102. Young KD. AMA seeks to protect residents from private equity career fallout. Available at: https://www.medscape.com/viewarticle/984503. Accessed January 25, 2023.

103. ACGME. Campbell University Program. Available at: https://apps.acgme-i.org/ads/Public/Programs/Detail?programId=32690. Accessed January 25, 2023.

104. Shanafelt TD, West CP, Dyrbye LN, et al. Changes in Burnout and Satisfaction With Work-Life Integration in Physicians During the First 2 Years of the COVID-19 Pandemic. Mayo Clin Proc 2022;97:2248–58.

105. Armona L, Chakrabarti R, Lovenheim MF. Student debt and default: the role of for-profit colleges. J Financ Econ 2022;144:67–92.

106. Robbins R. Medscape residents salary and debt report 2022. Available at: https://www.medscape.com/slideshow/2022-residents-salary-debt-report-6015490#9. Accessed January 25, 2023.

107. Gladwell M. Outliers: the story of success. 1st edition. New York, NY: Little, Brown and Company; 2008.

108. Cortez JL, Fadadu RP, Konda S, et al. Disparities in access for melanoma screening by region, specialty, and insurance: a cross-sectional audit study. JAAD Int 2022;7:78–85.

109. Novice T, Portney D, Eshaq M. Dermatology resident perspectives on practice ownership structures and private equity-backed group practices. Clin Dermatol 2020;38:296–302.

110. Hooke J. The Myth of private equity. New York, NY: Columbia University Press; 2021.

111. Scheffler RM, Alexander LM, Godwin JR. Soaring private equity investment in the healthcare sector: consolidation accelerated, competition undermined, and patients at risk. 2021. Available from: https://www.antitrustinstitute.org/wp-content/uploads/2021/05/Private-Equity-I-Healthcare-Report-FINAL.pdf. Accessed May 29, 2021.

112. Foerster J. Private equity heads south for a Riviera reality check. Available at: https://www.bloomberg.com/news/newsletters/2023-01-26/private-equity-heads-south-for-a-riviera-reality-check. Accessed January 25, 2023.

113. Farman M. Valuations top of mind as PE industry descends on cooler Cannes. Available at: https://www.privateequityinternational.com/valuations-top-of-mind-as-pe-industry-descends-on-cooler-cannes/. Accessed January 25, 2023.

114. International Private Equity Market. IPEM Cannes 2023. Available at: https://www.ipem-market.com/cannes-2023/. Accessed January 25, 2023.

115. Forefront Dermatology. 2023 Educational series. Available at: https://2023educationseries.rsvpify.com/. Accessed January 23, 2023.

116. Coldiron BM. Well, I figured it out. I owe my soul to the company store. Available at: https://www.mdedge.com/edermatologynews/article/152321/business-medicine/well-i-figured-it-out-i-owe-my-soul-company-store. Accessed January 25, 2023.

# Retirement Planning

Joshua Burshtein, MD[a,b,1], Danny Zakria, MD, MBA[a,b,*], Darrell Rigel, MD, MS[a,b]

**KEYWORDS**

- Retirement • Planning • Finance • Saving • Investment

**KEY POINTS**

- Retirement planning requires preparation for both financial and social aspects of life
- Understanding the benefits of retirement savings and the various plans available will give physicians the knowledge necessary to make informed decisions for financial planning
- Life after retirement also involves aspects outside of financial planning, something to provide meaning and purpose after work is complete

## INTRODUCTION

Planning for the future is required in all stages of life. There are several phases of a physician's career, each necessitating forward thinking. Beginning in college and medical school, then progressing to residency, early career and beyond, one critical component of daily practice is planning for the time after one's career is complete. The retirement process is an individualized endeavor, influenced by personal values as well as the surrounding environment.[1] In the 2018 Report on US Physicians' Financial Preparedness, the AMA found that 80% of retired physicians reported having a satisfying retirement.[2] As it is an important stage in one's life, retirement planning takes significant organization.

The process of retirement has been classified into three major stages: (a) preparation for retirement, (b) transitioning to retirement, and (c) adjusting to retirement.[3] The ability to successfully fulfill retirement plans is directly linked to retirement satisfaction.[4] At the point of retirement, individuals experience numerous changes at once, both financial and social, and it is important to understand the implications of these adjustments. When thinking about retirement planning, there are two main components, finances and quality of life. In this article, we discuss details of retirement planning, including the need to save, how much and when to start saving, types of retirement plans, and aspects of retirement outside of financial planning.

## DISCUSSION
### Should I Start Saving?

One of the first decisions in planning for financial retirement is to start saving money. It may be challenging to start saving for retirement at the beginning of a career, but setting a standard for allocating income to retire is beneficial for several reasons. Most obvious is the advantage of having financial resources to make retirement possible. Another benefit is the discipline which saving money entails. Being a lifelong endeavor, saving for retirement is a means for individuals to regulate spending practices in daily life and to maintain a lifestyle within their means.

Initial hesitancy to begin saving for retirement is natural. Prioritizing spending during residency/early career and waiting to save for retirement is a common mistake for physicians.[5] Disposable income is lower during these stages of life, but the financial penalty for missing out on accumulation of future wealth through investment makes this ideology problematic.[5] In general, the sooner you start saving, the better. Establishing contributions as early as residency can set the basis for future growth of wealth and provide a groundwork for retirement funds. From learning about financial markets and investment opportunities to benefiting

[a] National Society for Cutaneous Medicine, New York, NY, USA; [b] Department of Dermatology, Mount Sinai Icahn School of Medicine, 234 East 85th Street 5th Floor, New York, NY 10028, USA
[1] Present address: 1515 West 59th Street, New York, NY 10019, USA.
* Corresponding author. 234 East 85th Street 5th Floor, New York, NY 10028.
*E-mail address:* dzakria13@gmail.com

Dermatol Clin 41 (2023) 611–617
https://doi.org/10.1016/j.det.2023.05.006

from compound interest, beginning retirement saving early significantly increases your chances for a successful retirement.

This process starts by developing a financial budget, allocating a specific amount for savings, and initiating contributions to retirement-specific plans. As physicians transition to the early stages of their careers and especially as they progress throughout medical practice, ensuring thorough financial knowledge is key to successful retirement planning.

## How Much to Save?

Retirement saving is predicated on consistent allocation of income over the course of a career. The question then becomes, how much is needed to save? The answer, of course, varies based on each individual's goals. Factors that influence amount needed to save include lifestyle and anticipated spending rate during retirement, timing of retirement, projected life expectancy, and rate of inflation.[5] In 2014, Fidelity, a major financial institution, reported that the 5100 physicians in their records were predicted to replace only 56% of their income in retirement, saving about 15% of their yearly salary.[6] This was significantly under the recommended rate of 71% for those earning above $120,000 annually.[6] Per the Doximity 2023 Physician Compensation Report, dermatologists' average annual salary is $468,509.[7] Fidelity recommends people aim to save at least 15% of their income each year (including employer contributions) for retirement.[8]

The solution to determining how much to save is broken down into several parts. Estimating retirement needs can be accomplished by working backwards from anticipated future lifestyle, determining predicted expenses each retirement-year, and estimating the number of years in retirement.[5] To thoroughly understand the calculation for retirement savings, let us take an example (**Table 1**): a 32 year old dermatologist starting practice in 2023 who plans to retire at 65 year old. Assuming the present value of annual expenses of $100,000 in retirement and a life expectancy of 85 years,[9] the person would need to save $2,000,000 in present value. Yearly inflation must be taken into consideration and given a 33 year career (65 retirement age and age 32 at start of retirement saving), a physician needs to save an equivalent of $2,000,000 in 2056. If an inflation rate of 3% per year is assumed (based on historical estimates),[10] this would be an equivalent of $5,304,670 in 2056. Part of this dermatologist's savings will be in retirement accounts (401(k), 403(b), 457(b), Roth IRA, etc.), and the rest could

**Table 1**
**Example for calculation of retirement savings[a]**

| | |
|---|---|
| Retirement Age (Years) | 65 |
| Life expectancy age | 85 |
| Number of years in retirement | 20 |
| Present value of spending during retirement per annum | $100,000 |
| Total present value of spending needed during retirement (PV) | $2,000,000 |
| Rate of inflation per annum (r) | 3.00% |
| Age at which contributions to retirement plans begin | 32 |
| Retirement age | 65 |
| Number of years making contributions to retirement plans (n) | 33 |
| Formula calculating future value of savings needed during retirement | $FV = PV \times (1+r)^n$ |
| Future value of savings needed during retirement (FV) | $5,304,670 |
| Rate of return on retirement contributions per annum (R) | 5.00% |
| Number of years making contributions to retirement plans (n) | 33 |
| Formula calculating contributions to retirement plans per month (C) | $C = FV \times R/12/ ((1+R/12)^{(n \times 12)} - 1)$ |
| Contributions to retirement plans per month (C) | $5276 |
| Contributions to retirement plans per annum | $63,312 |

[a] The information is based on projected numbers and is provided for illustration purposes only. Calculations do not take into consideration employer matching contributions, social security benefits and taxes.

be in other investments. We will assume a 5% rate of return on investment.[11] This will require the dermatologist to contribute $5276 monthly ($63,312 per year) to retirement plans to achieve this financial retirement goal, representing 13.5% of dermatologists' average compensation. There are multiple websites that can provide you with these calculations as a starting point for your savings program (eg, https://www.investor.vanguard.com, https://www.bankrate.com, https://www.merrilledge.com).

## Plan for Retirement Saving

Retirement saving objectives can be successfully accomplished by establishing a well thought out strategy. A recent survey of academic physicians found that only 10% were satisfied with their retirement planning.[12] One of the primary reasons for such a low satisfaction rate is the lack of understanding of savings tools available for long-term financial planning.[12] As such, knowledge of retirement saving strategies is essential. The variety of retirement plans and savings opportunities can become overwhelming to those with a minimal wealth management background. It is important to analyze each type of retirement plan for its benefits and drawbacks and speak to a retirement specialist. A summary of the most common retirement plans is presented in **Table 2**.

Tax-advantaged savings accounts are a key component to the retirement portfolio.[5] The pre-

tax contributions to 401(k), 403(b), and 457(b) plans allow for a deferral of tax payments, and, consequently, for wealth growth on the higher invested capital. The tax is paid at the time of distribution, usually during retirement when the tax rates are lower.

An alternative option is to make after tax contributions to Roth 401(k) and 403(b) plans, with tax-free distributions taken at retirement.[13,14]

### Retirement Plans Available to Employees: 401(k), 403(b), 457(b) Plans

Dermatologists working for medical institutions should explore employer offered retirement plans and consider the employer's matching contribution when making decisions. For an employee, the 2023 annual combined employee and employer contributions are limited to $66,000 to all retirement accounts maintained by the employer.[8,15] The contribution limits are subject to cost-of-living adjustments in future years.

#### 401(k) plan
A common type of retirement plan that employees can contribute to is a 401(k), usually offered by for-profit companies. In 2023, the employee pretax contribution limit to a 401(k) is $22,500.

#### 403(b) plan
Tax-exempt organizations offer 403(b) plans that have similar contribution limits as 401(k) plans. In 2023, the employee pretax contribution limit to a 403(b) is $22,500.

#### 457(b) plan
Certain tax-exempt organizations establish 457(b) plans, where employees can contribute $22,500 in 2023. Employees working for not-for-profit institutions that offer both 403(b) and 457(b) plans can contribute $22,500 to each plan in 2023, for a total pretax contribution of $45,000.

### Employer Matching Contributions to 401(k), 403(b) Plans

Many employers provide matching contributions to 401(k) and 403(b) plans. The match amount is commonly 50% or 100% of the contribution made by the employee, and has a cap. The matching contributions usually have a vesting period, and the employee must be working for the employer for a specified number of years to garner full ownership of the employer contributions.

### Roth 401(k), Roth 403(b), Roth IRA Retirement Plans

Employees can choose to make after-tax contributions to either a Roth 401(k) or Roth 403(b)

| Table 2<br>Types of retirement plans and annual contribution limits for 2023[a] | |
| --- | --- |
| 401(k), 403(b) Defined contribution Plans | $22,500 |
| 475(b) defined compensation plan | $22,500 |
| Tax-exempt employers offering both 403(b) and 457(b) plans | $45,000 |
| Roth 401(k), 403(b) defined contribution plans | $22,500 |
| Roth IRA contribution plan | $6000 |
| Limit on annual contributions by employee to all plans at employer | $66,000 |
| SIMPLE 401(k) plan for self-employed | $15,500 |
| SEP (simplified employee pension) plan for self-employed | $66,000 |
| Defined benefit plan maximum contribution for self-employed | $265,000 |

[a] Most common retirement plans. A complete list can be found at https://www.irs.gov/retirement-plans/plan-sponsor/types-of-retirement-plans. The plan participation and contributions may be subject to additional restrictions. The contribution limits are determined by the Internal Revenue Service and are subject to cost-of-living adjustments in future years.

plan, whichever is offered by the employer, instead of making pre-tax contributions to 401(k) or 403(b) plans. Contributing to Roth retirement plans is advantageous when the income tax rates are expected to be higher in retirement as compared with the income tax rates during the years of employment. In 2023, employee contribution to employer-sponsored Roth retirement plans is limited to $22,500.

Individuals can also set up and contribute to a Roth IRA. Contributions are limited to $6000 in 2023, and fully phase out at modified Adjusted Gross Income (MAGI) in excess of $218,000 for the taxpayer status of married filing jointly, and in excess of $138,000 for all other taxpayers.

Roth IRAs provide for tax exempt growth, tax exempt withdrawals, and these benefits may be available to your heirs. This makes them the most valuable retirement vehicle for most physicians. Note there currently still is a "backdoor" Roth IRA for individuals making over the MAGI. If an individual makes an after tax contribution of up to $6000 to a conventional IRA, this can be converted (as soon as the following day) to a Roth IRA on a yearly basis.

In addition, conventional IRAs can be converted whole or in part to a Roth by paying the income tax that would have been due at the time of the roll over. This can be a useful strategy when the value of your conventional IRA is greatly depressed by a market downturn.

### Retirement Plans Available to Private Practice and Self-employed: SIMPLE 401(k), simplified employee pension IRA, Defined Benefit Plan, Money Purchase Plan, Profit Sharing Plan

For physicians who own their own practice, there are multiple plans and diverse saving opportunities including SIMPLE 401(k), simplified employee pension (SEP) IRA, defined benefit plan, money purchase plan, and profit-sharing plan. The choice for the appropriate retirement savings plans depends on specific situations. Some of the factors to consider when selecting a retirement plan are the costs associated with the administration of retirement plans, the number of employees, and the profitability of the practice.

### SIMPLE 401(k) plan

A SIMPLE 401(k) plan is for employers with 100 or fewer employees. It is similar to a 401(k) plan, with a notable difference that the employer must make either a matching contribution up to 3% of each employee's pay, or a non-elective contribution of 2% of each eligible employee's salary.[14]

### SEP IRA plan

A SEP IRA plan allows for a contribution of up to 25% of each employee's compensation, up to a maximum of $66,000 for 2023.[16,17] One of the benefits of this plan is the lack of start-up and operating costs.

### Defined Benefit Plan

A defined benefit plan provides for a predictable monthly benefit at retirement. The retirement payment is based on factors such as the participant's salary, age, and number of years working for the employer. Under this plan, the annual maximum contribution by the employer is the lesser of the participant's average compensation for 3 consecutive calendar years or $265,000 for 2023. A defined benefit plan allows employers to contribute substantially more than other retirement plans; however, there are minimum contribution requirements and operating costs must be considered as this is the most administratively complex plan.

### Money Purchase Plan

A money purchase plan requires a fixed percentage (specified in the plan) of income contribution annually up to 25% of compensation, with a contribution limit of $66,000 for 2023.[16]

### Profit-Sharing Plan

A profit-sharing plan allows the employer to decide how much to contribute annually up to 25% of compensation, with a contribution limit of $66,000 for 2023.

### Investment Strategies

Once retirement plans are selected and contribution amounts determined, physicians should consider investment strategies. In general terms, there are 3 main investment strategies: conservative, hybrid, and very aggressive—and there is a varying degree of risk associated with each. Conservative risk strategies recommend investing in low-volatility assets, such as short-term bonds and bank certificates of deposit, and are generally utilized by those closer to retirement age. The further a person is from retirement age, the more attractive an aggressive investment strategy becomes, concentrating in volatile assets with high-risk/return attributes. A hybrid strategy advocates for an investment portfolio comprised low- and high-volatile assets. A recommended approach is to develop an asset allocation strategy whereby retirement savings are split among multiple asset classes (ie, stock, bonds, commodities, etc.) to reduce the risk of being too heavily concentrated in one type of investment.[5,13] If the investment options offered by the plans are overwhelming, choose a target-date fund aligned with your anticipated year of retirement. If you do not feel that you are knowledgeable in the investment space, it is recommended that a financial consultant's guidance is utilized for investment advice.

## When to Retire?

The timing of retirement for physicians depends on a variety of factors. From lifestyle preference and financial preparedness to gratification with work and desire to maintain work identity, the determinants for retirement vary from person to person. A systematic review found that the most commonly reported age of physician retirement was between 60 and 69 years of age.[18] Most physicians remained in practice past the typical retirement age of 65 years.[18] In a national survey, age of retirement across all medical specialties between 2001 and 2009 increased from 64 to 66.5 years.[19] Regarding dermatologists specifically, average age of retirement rose from 61 years in 2007 to 65.5 years in 2009.[19] The reason for this is not one-dimensional but includes financial as well as social incentives. Physicians, just like the general public, may be concerned about the financial security that a job provides. As such, retirement planning is essential to a smooth transition to retirement.

The decision for when to retire is a significant one. With this decision comes a change in daily routine and a separation from the practice of medicine that physicians have been dedicated to for decades. The work environment provides structure, community, and purpose, and retirement may bring with it a loss of identity and unstructured routine.[20] In a survey study of chairs of academic ophthalmology departments, 16% of chairs said excessive leisure time was the major source of anxiety for retirement.[21]

Retirement planning may not always go as expected. Unexpected circumstances are likely to arise, most significant of which may be health related. Spending too much on lifestyle expenses, periods of unemployment, funding children's education, caring for loved ones, and other factors can also contribute to falling behind on retirement savings.

Those that choose to retire early may do so due to challenges in their professional and personal lives. Factors such as financial constraints, poor job satisfaction, and health concerns can all play a role. In the workplace, excessive workload, burnout, feeling undervalued, and loss of interest in work have all been documented as reasons for early retirement.[18] On the other hand, those who delay retirement may do so for financial reasons, satisfaction with their work, commitment to patient care, and continued intellectual stimulation.[18]

The ultimate decision of when to retire is related to a multitude of variables but should be viewed as a transition rather than a specific day. For some, working part-time may be a means to slowly transition to retirement. Ultimately, if one does not feel ready for retirement, then it is not the time to retire. Practicing medicine for many years brings with it meaning and purpose, and it is essential to also focus on these aspects of life when planning for retirement.

## Other Considerations for Retirement Planning

Financial planning is only one component of preparation for retirement. To have a successful retirement, one must have something to retire to. The transition to retirement necessitates redefining purpose and finding meaningful activities to fill the void of work. This process requires drive and creativity to be productive with one's free time.[20] Determining what derives meaning from daily life, whether that be family and friends or hobbies such as sports, arts, travel, or volunteerism, can help prevent negative emotions that may come with retirement.

One study found that after 5 years into retirement, 40% of individuals experienced boredom or sadness, and felt happier prior to retiring.[22] After working for decades and planning for financial stability for retirement, why does this occur? For physicians, daily work provides purpose, passion, status, and the ability to positively impact the lives of others. Retirement must therefore replace these aspects of fulfillment. Without the need to focus on acquisition,[22] retirement allows for a shift to desires outside of money or materials. Increased efforts on volunteering or philanthropy are ways to be productive that can also provide a sense of purpose. During a physician's career, discovering interests outside of work are vital, whether that be in medicine, education, or other domains, and these interests can be continued throughout retirement.

Other factors that contribute to a meaningful life in retirement are maintaining one's health and relationships. A survey of retired orthopedic surgeons showed predictors for postretirement satisfaction included health and a better relationship with one's spouse.[23] Friends and family are a support system that may matter even more during

**Box 1**
**Retirement Strategy for Dermatologists**

1. *Start early:* The earlier you start planning for your retirement, the more time you have to save and invest. Dermatologists should begin planning for their retirement as soon as possible, ideally in their early 20s or 30s.

2. *Determine your retirement goals:* Before you can plan for retirement, you need to know what your retirement goals are. Dermatologists should consider factors such as the lifestyle they want to maintain in retirement, the age at which they want to retire, and their expected expenses in retirement.

3. *Calculate your retirement income needs:* Once you know your retirement goals, you can calculate how much income you will need to achieve them. Dermatologists should consider factors such as social security benefits, pensions, and any other sources of retirement income.

4. *Maximize your retirement contributions:* Dermatologists should take advantage of retirement accounts such as 401(k)s, IRAs, and other retirement savings plans. Maximize your contributions to these accounts each year to save as much as possible.

5. *Diversify your investments:* Investing in a diverse range of assets can help protect your retirement savings from market fluctuations. Dermatologists should consider investing in a mix of stocks, bonds, and other assets to achieve a diversified portfolio.

6. *Consider working with a financial advisor:* A financial advisor can provide valuable guidance and advice on retirement planning. Dermatologists should work with a financial advisor to develop a comprehensive retirement plan that takes into account their unique needs and goals.

retirement, as more time is available to spend with loved ones.

## SUMMARY

Retirement planning and saving provides financial resources to ensure a high quality of life during retirement. The key to a successful retirement is careful planning (**Box 1**) and the right attitude, something that cannot be influenced by anyone but the individual. Retirement is not a time when life stops; rather, it is an exciting period that allows for exploring new adventures, continuing lifelong passions and relationships, and enjoying the financial stability that has been planned for after years of hard work.

## CLINICS CARE POINTS

Plan to maximize financial resources and satisfaction in retirement.

- Start contributing to retirement saving plans as early as possible
- Make maximum allowed contributions
- Understand different investment options and select the approach to meet objectives
- Consider qualitative attributes for life in retirement: maintaining good health, time with friends and family, volunteering, philanthropy, and hobbies

## DISCLOSURE

J. Burshtein, MD has no conflicts to disclose. D. Zakria, MD, MBA has no conflicts to disclose. D. Rigel, MD MS has no conflicts to disclose.

## REFERENCES

1. Cahill KE, Giandrea MD, Quinn JF. Retirement Patterns and the Macroeconomy, 1992–2010: The Prevalence and Determinants of Bridge Jobs, Phased Retirement, and Reentry Among Three Recent Cohorts of Older Americans. Gerontol 2015;55(3):384–403.
2. Farouk A. 6 key physician retirement insights from doctors already there. Published online November 8, 2018. https://www.ama-assn.org/practice-management/career-development/6-key-physician-retirement-insights-doctors-already-there. Accessed April 23, 2023.
3. Hewitt A, Howie L, Feldman S. Retirement: What will you do? A narrative inquiry of occupation-based planning for retirement: Implications for practice. Aust Occup Ther J 2010;57(1):8–16.
4. Principi A, Smeaton D, Cahill K, et al. What Happens to Retirement Plans, and Does This Affect Retirement Satisfaction? Int J Aging Hum Dev 2020;90(2):152–75.
5. Turin SY, Fine P, Fine N. Wealth Management and Retirement. Plast Reconstr Surg 2022;149(2):323e–32e.
6. Stewart J. Budgeting for retirement: make a plan and stick to it. Med Econ 2015;92(23):46–51.
7. 2023 Physician Compensation Report. https://press.doximity.com/reports/doximity-physician-compensation-report-2023.pdf. Accessed April 23, 2023.
8. Fidelity Smart Money. 401(k) contribution limits 2022 and 2023. Fidelity. Published December 15, 2022. https://www.fidelity.com/learning-center/smart-money/401k-contribution-limits. Accessed April 24, 2023.

9. Medina L, Sabo S, Vespa J. "Living Longer: Historical and Projected Life Expectancy in the United States, 1960 to 2060." Current Population Reports, Available at: www.census.gov/content/dam/Census/library/publications/2020/demo/p25-1145.pdf. Accessed April 23, 2023.

10. Inflation expectations. Federal Reserve Bank of Cleveland. https://www.clevelandfed.org/indicators-and-data/inflation-expectations. Accessed April 24, 2023.

11. Our investment and economic forecasts, January 2023. Vanguard. Published January 2023. https://corporate.vanguard.com/content/corporatesite/us/en/corp/articles/investment-economic-outlook-january-2023.html. Accessed April 24, 2023.

12. Pannor Silver M, Easty LK. Planning for retirement from medicine: a mixed-methods study. CMAJ Open 2017;5(1):E123–9.

13. Treiger TM. Retirement—If You Fail to Plan, Then You Plan to Fail. Prof Case Manag 2016;21(1):43–5.

14. 401(k) plan overview. Internal Revenue Service. https://www.irs.gov/retirement-plans/plan-sponsor/401k-plan-overview. Accessed April 24, 2023.

15. 401(k) limit increases to $22,500 for 2023, IRA limit rises to $6,500. Internal Revenue Service. https://www.irs.gov/newsroom/401k-limit-increases-to-22500-for-2023-ira-limit-rises-to-6500. Accessed April 24, 2023.

16. Retirement plans for self-employed people. Internal Revenue Service. https://www.irs.gov/retirement-plans/retirement-plans-for-self-employed-people. Accessed April 24, 2023.

17. Nabity J. Everything you need to know about physician retirement. Physicians Thrive. Published October 20, 2022. https://physiciansthrive.com/retirement-planning/physicians-need-know. Accessed April 24, 2023.

18. Silver MP, Hamilton AD, Biswas A, et al. A systematic review of physician retirement planning. Hum Resour Health 2016;14(1):67.

19. Dermatologists more likely to delay retirement. Dermatology Times. Published May 1, 2010. https://www.dermatologytimes.com/view/dermatologists-more-likely-delay-retirement. Accessed April 22, 2023.

20. Cronan JJ. Retirement: It's Not About the Finances. J Am Coll Radiol 2009;6(4):242–5.

21. Dodds DW, Cruz OA, Israel H. Attitudes toward Retirement of Ophthalmology Department Chairs. Ophthalmology 2013;120(7):1502–5.

22. Bernstein A, Trauth J. Your retirement, your way: why it takes more than money to live your Dream. New York: McGraw-Hill; 2007.

23. Ritter M, Austrom M, Zhou H, et al. Retirement from orthopaedic surgery. J Bone Joint Surg Am 1999;81:414 – 8. J Bone Jt Surg 1999;81:414–8.

# Expanding and Strengthening Your Referral Network

Payvand Kamrani, DO[a], Alexandra Flamm, MD[b],*

## KEYWORDS

- Referrals • Communication • MIPS • Teledermatology • Coding • Social media

## KEY POINTS

- Referral utilization has increased over the decades with 15% of dermatology-related visits by primary care resulting in a dermatology referral.
- Effective communication between specialist and referring provider is essential for efficient and high-level patient-oriented coordinated care.
- Written and/or verbal communication with referring providers can help build a strong communication network and, in some instances, can be applied towards Merit-based Incentive Payment System (MIPS) reporting.
- Reaching out directly to referring clinics directly has been shown to increase the quantity of referrals, including providing clinics patient handouts, education on what information to prioritize in referrals, and how to complete referrals effectively and efficiently.
- Social media plays a major role in referrals, especially for patients looking for cosmetic care. There are many different platforms and can serve as a marketing tool for physicians looking to bring in new patients.

## BACKGROUND

Referrals are an important part of a dermatology practice's patient base and they have overall been increasing. Studies have shown referral rates to dermatologists nearly doubled from 1999 to 2009.[1,2] In 2006 to 2009, 15% of visits to a primary care physician resulted in a dermatology referral.[1]

This increase in dermatology referrals may be due to several reasons, including a relative lack of dermatology training in medical school training, malpractice concerns, and patient preference.[2] Referrals can add to unnecessary expenditures within the health care system, with one study noting a referral can cost roughly six times more than appropriate initial treatment.[3] Therefore a nuanced discussion regarding need for referral is important. Here we discuss strategies to both strengthen and expand the referral network of dermatologists.

### Effective communication

Communication between primary care physicians (PCPs) and specialists regarding referrals is often inadequate and inconsistent, which can result in negative consequences for the patient, including delays in diagnosis, unnecessary testing, iatrogenic complications, and polypharmacy.[4,5]

For example, Stille and colleagues found that specialists reported communicating with referring providers only 50% of the time, with the most common barriers including not enough personnel, lack of skills, and not enough time.[6] A national physician survey in 2008 of 4720 physicians noted that 69% of PCPs reported always or most of the

[a] Department of Dermatology, Penn State Health, 200 Campus Drive, Suite 100, Hershey, PA 17033, USA;
[b] Department of Dermatology, NYU Grossman School of Medicine, 222 East 41st Street, 25th Floor, New York, NY 10017, USA
* Corresponding author. NYU Department of Dermatology, 222 East 41st Street, 25th Floor, New York, NY 10017.
E-mail address: alexandra.flamm@nyulangone.org

Dermatol Clin 41 (2023) 619–626
https://doi.org/10.1016/j.det.2023.06.001

time sending notification of a patient's history and reason for consultation to the specialists, however, only 34% of specialists said they received such notifications.[7] Only 80% of referring physicians reported they received consultation reports from specialists always or most of the time post-visit.[7] This survey also found that physicians who do not receive a timely communication regarding the outcome of a referral were more likely to report that their ability to perform high-quality care was threatened.[7] This review also analyzed factors that were associated with improved communication outcomes, which included more time for administrative tasks and having staff to coordinate care.[7,8]

### Strategies to improve communication

A standardized referral letter can offer clear and concise information about a patient to aid the specialist and reduce unnecessary repetition of care or delayed diagnosis. Standardized referral letters should include patient's names, symptoms, diagnostic results, treatments given, co-morbidities, significant family history, and most importantly, reason for referral. See **Box 1** for an example of a standardized referral letter. A

standardized reply form can also be included to aid in quickly and efficiently conveying information from the consultation to the patient and their referring provider (**Box 2**).

Regardless of the template used, a structured letter with headings has been shown to enhance the quality of referrals.[9] However as previously noted, time constrains and lack of ancillary support have been cited as reasons for sub-optimal referral letters.[10,11] Additionally, these letters may not necessarily lead to an improvement in follow up communication between specialists and referring providers.[9]

Given the time-intensive nature of ensuring effective communication, appropriate reimbursement is imperative. However, difficulty can arise in ensuring appropriate reimbursement for the coordination of care. There are several care coordination common procedural terminology (Trademarked CPT) codes; however, these can only be utilized under very specific circumstances. The chronic care management code 99490, for instance, can only be utilized when at least 20 minutes of clinical staff time occurs under the direction of physician or qualified health care provider per calendar month. In order to bill this code, the patient must have at least two chronic conditions that are expected to last at least 1 year,

---

**Box 1**
**Standardized referral letter**

Date

Standard Referral Letter

Reason for referral: _____

_____

Patient Name: _____  Age: ____  MRN: _____

Past Medical History: _____

_____

Current Medications: _____  Allergies: _____

Clinical Presentation: _____

Lab and Imaging Studies: _____

Probable Diagnosis: _____

Treatments tried and reason for failure: _____

_____

Additional pertinent information: _____

_____

Thank you,

Dr. *Referring Physican*
P: 555-555-5555 F: 555-555-55555

---

**Box 2**
**Formatted referral response**

PRACTICE OR PHYSICIAN'S NAME
Address | Telephone | Email

Date

Dr. *Referring Physician*
Title
Company
Street Address
City, ST ZIP Code

Dear Dr. *Referring Physician*:

Thank you for your referral for [Patient's Name], who was referred to me on [Referral Date] for [Reason for Referral]. After a thorough examination and review of [Patient's name] history, we have reached a probable diagnosis of [diagnosis].

The following next steps include:

- [List any orders including laboratory evaluation, imaging, or any new or adjusted medications]

Follow up:

- [List follow up plan]

Instructions for referring physicians:

- [List any further instructions for the referring physicians]

Please notify me of any changes or additional information that becomes available. If you have any questions or concerns, please do not hesitate to contact me.

Sincerely,

Practice or physician's name

or until the death of the patient. In addition, these conditions place the patient at a significant risk of death, acute exacerbation/decompensation, or functional decline.[12] An example could include a patient with flaring systemic lupus erythematosus and symptomatic anemia, for which coordination with the patient's rheumatologist and hematologist is necessary.

If the physician does the care coordination directly, such as speaking with the patient's other providers to ensure appropriate follow-up visits and treatments, there is also a possibility this care could be incorporated into the billing for an associated Evaluation & Management (E/M) visit, as long as other care coordination codes are not being simultaneously utilized.[12] This can be incorporated into billing either by time or medical decision making (MDM).

When billing by time, care coordination performed by the physician directly on the day of the encounter can be included in the total time used to determine the level of an E/M visit. For example, you see a patient for pemphigus vulgaris, notice they have worsening dysphagia, and then contact their gastroenterologist directly after the visit, spending 10 minutes discussing these symptoms and arranging for further testing. These 10 minutes of time can be included in the total time of the E/M performed that day. Importantly your documentation should include this discussion and the time it encompassed. Staff time spent on the coordination of care cannot be counted here.[13]

When billing by MDM, physician-to-physician communication is specifically incorporated within the AMA MDM billing table. For example, you see a patient with psoriasis and worsening joint pain who is taking methotrexate and then call the patient's rheumatologist to discuss modifications to the patient's systemic treatments. This discussion would meet the moderate level in the second column of the MDM table (Amount and/or Complexity of Data to be Reviewed and Analyzed).[13]

The AMA does have guidelines regarding the definition of "discussion." Specifically, this must be a direct interactive exchange, and not through intermediaries (eg, clinical staff or trainees). Sending chart notes or written exchanges that are within progress notes does not qualify. For MDM, the discussion does not need to be on the date of the encounter and can be asynchronous, but must be initiated and completed within a short time period (eg, 1–2 days). The discussion is also counted only once and only when it is used in the decision making of the encounter.[13]

Communication between specialist and referring provider can also be applied toward Merit-based Incentive Payment System (MIPS) reporting. There are three MIPS outcomes in particular that can be reported related to this type of communication: MIPS 138, 265, 364 (Table 1).[14]

Melanoma: Coordination of Care (MIPS 138), looks at the percentage of patient visits with a new diagnosis of melanoma that have a documented treatment plan communicated to the primary physician or physician responsible for continuing care. This plan must be communicated within 1 month of the diagnosis, regardless of the patient's age. Biopsy Follow Up (MIPS 265), looks at the percentage of new patients whose biopsy results have been shared with both the referring physician and the patient. Lastly, Closing the Referral Loop (MIPS 374) looks at the percentage of patients with referrals who had their referring provider receive a report from the provider they were referred to.[14]

Effective communication between dermatologists and dermatopathologists is also critical in providing high-quality patient care. The clinical history on the pathology requisition form is often the only communication between dermatologists and pathologists. As a dermatologist, consistently providing relevant and precise information can help decrease turnaround time, insufficient sampling, and increase the use of stains.[15,16] Include a brief differential diagnosis, clinical description, significant comorbidities, and prior biopsies, if applicable. For inflammatory diseases, description, duration, and prior treatments can be useful. For neoplastic lesions, size and location can assist with staging. This relationship is fundamental in sustaining a well-run practice.[17] See **Box 3** for an example of an effective requisition form.

## Expanding physician-based referrals

Reaching out directly to nearby referring practices has been shown to increase referral numbers.[18] However, lack of understanding from the referring office on how to initiate the referral and lack of knowledge on appropriate referral criteria have been cited as common barriers to the direct referral process. Therefore, a tailored approach to individual practice regions and physician composition is important to ensuring a robust referral network. An emphasis on interacting with referring practices in-person is of particular use.

For example, a high-risk skin cancer clinic was looking to better understand their referral network. The group conducted in-person visits to five of their high-volume referring clinics in order to answer any questions the referring clinics had, providing newly developed educational materials, as well as a step-by-step guide on making

**Table 1**
**MIPS Report codes for incentivizing communication**

| MIPS Number | Description | How is it calculated | Maximum number of points |
|---|---|---|---|
| MIPS 138 Melanoma: Coordination of Care | The percentage of patient visits with a new diagnosis of melanoma that have a documented treatment plan, which was communicated to the physician(s) responsible for continuing care, within 1 month of the diagnosis, regardless of the patient's age. | *The numerator:* the number of patients with a new diagnosis of melanoma who had their treatment plan communicated to the physicians responsible for continuing care. *The denominator:* the total number of patients with a new diagnosis of melanoma | 7 |
| MIPS 265 Biopsy Follow up | The percentage of new patients whose biopsy results have been reviewed and shared with both the primary care/referring physician and the patient. | *The numerator:* the number of patients whose biopsy results were shared with the primary care physician or referring physician. *The denominator:* the total number of new patients who underwent a biopsy. | 7 |
| MIPS 374 Closing the Referral Loop | The percentage of patients with referrals, regardless of age, who had their referring provider receive a report from the provider they were referred to. | *The numerator:* the number of patients with referrals during the reporting period whose referring physician received a report back. *The denominator:* the total number of new patients who were referred by another provider during the reporting period. | 10 |

referrals. Following this intervention, the average number of monthly referrals increased from 11.9 to 25.2 in less than 1 year.[18]

Local or state-run conferences and/or meetings, such as local medical society meetings are also another way to meet local physicians. This can allow for opportunities for cross-specialty networking and thus creating working relationships.

### Wait times and referral networks

Ensuring reasonable wait times for new referrals is also important when expanding a referral network. Having a longer wait time for new appointments may discourage referring physicians from sending referrals. Telehealth for initial visits can often be an effective tool to help decrease wait times. For example, at San Francisco General Hospital, a new referral system required all referrals undergoes an electronic specialist review which allowed the clinic to address 20% of PCP-initiated referrals through electronic messaging alone.[2,19,20]

A similar study was done by Tang and colleagues analyzing gastroenterology referrals. This group reviewed all electronic referrals for 5 months prior to scheduling and conducted an electronic consultation. Of the 1243 electronic referrals reviewed, only 29% resulted in a clinic appointment. Many resolved without a need for the clinic visit and many were able to be directly scheduled for their procedure without a clinic appointment.[21]

---

**Box 3**
Example dermatopathology requisition form

**Dermatopathology Lab Requisition Form**

Requesting physician name: _____

Requesting physician contact information: _____


Patient name: _____

Patient date of birth: _____

Patient medical record number: _____

[ ] Female [ ] Male


Procedure:_____       _____

Specimen site:_____

Clinical history:_____

Clinical diagnosis:_____

Special requests:_____

Previous biopsies:_____

---

This can be applicable in dermatology for example, with patients with a biopsy-proven skin cancer who need to be referred for a surgery excision. Scheduling the patient directly for a surgery appointment can open a clinic appointment for another new referral and is more convenient for the patients.

Creating a restricted referral list may help with improving wait times for new referrals. Many dermatology clinics in the United Kingdom, for example, have created a restricted-referral list to improve wait times for new referrals, specifically due to governmental pressures to meet strict requirements on skin cancer waiting time.[22] Some studies have also proposed the use of patient-report outcomes to help expedite referral. A UK clinic required referrals to include a Dermatology Life Quality Index Score (DLQI) and used this score to triage patients with psoriasis for more urgent referral appointments.[23] Restricted referral lists may however deter some referring providers from placing referrals and therefore may not be as useful when looking to expand a referral network.

### Barriers to physician-based referrals

Previously, reaching out to colleagues to encourage referrals was common. However, this practice of direct referral has decreased due to constraints, such as health insurance and health system requirements, as well as increasing wait times for appointments. An increase in consolidation within medicine has accelerated this trend,

requiring physicians to refer to specialists within particular health systems.[24] The COVID-19 pandemic has also accelerated the process of consolidation, with an increasing number of physician practice transaction occurring after the onset of the pandemic when compared to prior.[25] This trend is not only specific to dermatology, but also seen in many fields of medicine, including ophthalmology, rheumatology, and primary care.[26]

### Social media and expanding patient-based referrals

A referral incentive program can help motivate current patients to refer your practice to family and friends. Providing a reward to existing customers is used routinely outside of medicine and incentives include cash, store discounts, or specific brand discounts.[27] However, in our review, we found no strong evidence that a referral incentive program in medicine increased referrals.

Social media has become an accessible and popular avenue for networking and outreach in dermatology, especially among younger age groups and those seeking cosmetic treatments.[28,29] Although thought be a tool specific to the younger generation, new data has also demonstrated that nearly 50% of individuals above the age of 65 use social media.[29]

In 2018, it was estimated that 3 billion out of the 7.7 billion population uses at least one form of social media.[28] However while 80% of patients use the internet to search for medication information, only 15% of dermatologists utilize social media for professional reasons.[29]

There are many different platforms including Meta (formerly Facebook), Twitter, Instagram, Tik-Tok, YouTube, Snapchat, and other emerging platforms. Dermatologists can benefit from these platforms via opportunities for connection and engagement with current and future patients as well as colleagues. For example, dermatologic journals such as the *Journal of American Academy of Dermatology,* and residency programs have also increased their presence over the past 5 years, increasing opportunities for networking and education.[28]

Some social media platforms can also assess the impact of your engagement with users on their platforms and the effectiveness of your interventions, for example, by evaluating referrals to your website directly from social media sites.[30] Meta offers "Facebook insights" which can provide the user with weekly total reach, and detailed ways to monitor audience and outreach.

Patients use social media for numerous purposes including referral services.[29,30] A survey of a cosmetic dermatology practice found that about 15% of their patients were self-referred to their clinic due to their high social media presence. Additionally, multiple studies note that many patients look to social media more than television or print advertisements in finding a dermatologist, with those seeking dermatologic care for medical purposes preferring Twitter and those seeking cosmetic treatments preferring Instagram.[30,31]

**Table 2**
**Common social media platforms**

|  | General Use | Dermatology Use |
| --- | --- | --- |
| Facebook | Self-produced content with personalized profile; ability to directly message; business profiles can connect with customers, advertise products and service, build brand awareness | • Ability to create a business page to share information about practice, location, hours of operation, types of services offered.<br>• Facebook ads offer targeted advertising options to reach specific audiences<br>• Sharing dermatology educational content to establish yourself as an expert |
| Instagram | Similar to Facebook with individual profiles and messaging service however allows the ability to search content through hashtags; visual platform which allows for videos, reels, photos to be shared | • Instagram stories allow for short photos and videos which can be used for educational content new products or services<br>• Hashtag use can help expand to a wider audience by using relevant dermatology and trending hashtags |
| Tik-Tok | Social Media platform with unique short clip videos with the ability to share audio to different users | • Ability to create short videos about skin conditions and treatments |
| Twitter | Allows users to create and share short comments called "tweets" with similar engagement to Instagram with hashtags | • Ability to post articles, posts, and reliable information about dermatology conditions<br>• Using tags by "@user" to engage industry and experts in the field, which then can be sharedtheir follows to increase the spread of content |

Joining Facebook Groups for specific diagnoses can also be an effective way to connect with possible patients, in particular, if you have a specialty clinic or an interest in that specific field. For example, the largest online support group for patients with hidradenitis suppurative (HS) is on Facebook with over 15,000 members to date. **Table 2** reviews different social media platforms in further detail.

Increasing engagement on social media platforms can pose a challenge. The first step is to consider who is the target audience and increase posts and content tailored to this group. Physicians can utilize Google Alerts, which allow them to receive e-mail updates for commonly searched google inquires. This can help monitor what dermatology-related trends may be on social media at the time and create postings that incorporate these topics.[29] The use of trending hashtags on many social media platforms can help with increasing outreach. Staff support for social media is important given the need to post frequent updates on these platforms. Some offices have even created a social media content creator position.

Despite its potential benefits, there are some risks to the use of social media including the inadvertently posting protected health information, as well as security concerns.[32] Surveyed physicians indicated the top reason for not interacting with patients through a social media platform were liability and privacy concerns.[33] Additionally responses to a single follower can be disseminated and distributed to numerous other users where the advice is not applicable. Therefore, it is important to place a disclaimer on a physicians' social media pages stating they do not provide medical advice through this platform.

### Telemedicine

Teledermatology has been utilized as a method of delivering dermatologic care remotely to patients. It has been transformed following the emergence of the COVID-19 pandemic in which many dermatologic practices were closed due to social distancing restrictions. Asynchronous, or store-and-forward teledermatology, involves the transfer of medical information and photos for a dermatologist at a different location to review at a time when the patient is not present. Synchronous teledermatology, on the other hand, usually involves face-to-face video conferencing allowing real-time interactions.[34] Telehealth has the potential to significantly reduce patient wait time for evaluation to treatment and improve overall patient access by increasing the number of patients that can be evaluated.

Telemedicine has shown promise in increasing efficient post-operative care, eliminating a significant number of unnecessary referrals, and connecting patients that may be far from large health-care facilities.[35] Telemedicine has been consistently rated as convenient and easy for patients, referring physicians, and consulting dermatologists. However, despite a major increase in teledermatology use following the COVID pandemic, there is a paucity of evidence-based studies evaluating referral numbers following implementing telehealth into a dermatology practice.

## SUMMARY

Different techniques can be utilized to help expand and strengthen a practice's referral network. Effective communication is a key component, and there are now multiple ways to incorporate the coordination of care into the reimbursement structure of E/M visits. Reaching out to nearby referring practices and the incorporation of social media can also aid in expanding referral networks. Telehealth may help reach individuals who may not otherwise visit a practice due to location, however, its use with increasing referrals has not yet been fully evaluated.

## CLINICS CARE POINTS

- Effective communication between specialist and referring provider is essential for efficient and high-level patient-oriented coordinated care.

- Written and verbal communication can in some instances be applied towards Merit-based Incentive Payment System (MIPS) reporting and requirements for coordination of care coding.

- Reaching out directly to referring clinics directly has been shown to increase the quantity of referrals.

- Social media plays a major role in referrals and can serve as a marketing tool for physicians looking to bring in new patients.

## DISCLOSURE

None reported.

## CONFLICTS OF INTEREST

None reported.

## REFERENCES

1. Barnett ML, Keating NL, Christakis NA, et al. Reasons for choice of referral physician among primary care and specialist physicians. J Gen Intern Med 2012;27(5):506–12.

2. Song Z, Rose S, Safran DG, et al. Changes in health care spending and quality 4 years into global payment. N Engl J Med 2014;371(18):1704–14.

3. Sladden M, Graham-Brown R. How many GP referrals to dermatology outpatients are really necessary? J R Soc Med 1989;82(6):347–8.

4. O'Malley AS, Reschovsky JD. Referral and consultation communication between primary care and specialist physicians: finding common ground. Arch Intern Med 2011;171(1):56–65.

5. Ramanayake R. Structured printed referral letter (form letter); saves time and improves communication. J Fam Med Prim Care 2013;2(2):145.

6. Stille CJ, McLaughlin TJ, Primack WA, et al. Determinants and impact of generalist–specialist communication about pediatric outpatient referrals. Pediatrics 2006;118(4):1341–9.

7. Lee D, Begley CE. Physician report of industry gifts and quality of care. Health Care Manag Rev 2016; 41(3):275–83.

8. Deshpande SP, DeMello J. A comparative analysis of factors that hinder primary care physicians' and specialist physicians' ability to provide high-quality care. Health Care Manag 2011;30(2):172–8.

9. Couper I, Henbest R. The quality and relationship of referral and reply letters. S Afr Med J 1996;86(12): 1540–2.

10. Karunarathna LDA. Consulting wisely-an art in family medicine. Sri Lankan Family Physician 1999;22:8–15.

11. Gandhi TK, Sittig DF, Franklin M, et al. Communication breakdown in the outpatient referral process. J Gen Intern Med 2000;15(9):626–31.

12. Coding and Billing for Care Coordination. 2018.

13. CPT E/M Office Revisions Level of Medical Decision Making (MDM). 2021.

14. 2022 QUALITY MEASURES FOR MIPS REPORTING.

15. Romano RC, Novotny PJ, Sloan JA, et al. Measures of completeness and accuracy of clinical information in skin biopsy requisition forms: an analysis of 249 cases. Am J Clin Pathol 2016;146(6):727–35.

16. Comfere NI, Peters MS, Jenkins S, et al. Dermatopathologists' concerns and challenges with clinical information in the skin biopsy requisition form: a mixed-methods study. J Cutan Pathol 2015;42(5):333–45.

17. Smith SD, Reimann JD, Horn TD. Communication Between Dermatologists and Dermatopathologists via the Pathology Requisition: Opportunities to Improve Patient Care. JAMA dermatology 2021;157(9):1033–4.

18. Weintraub GS, Su KA, Demehri S, et al. Enhancing the process for care delivery in a dermatology specialty clinic. J Am Acad Dermatol 2020;83(4):1181–4.

19. Kim-Hwang JE, Chen AH, Bell DS, et al. Evaluating electronic referrals for specialty care at a public hospital. J Gen Intern Med 2010;25(10):1123–8. https://doi.org/10.1007/s11606-010-1402-1.

20. Cotton VR. Legal risks of "curbside" consults. Am J Cardiol 2010;106:135–8.

21. Tang Z, Dubois S, Soon C, et al. A model for the pandemic and beyond: Telemedicine for all outpatient gastroenterology referrals reduces unnecessary clinic visits. J Telemed Telecare 2022;28(8): 577–82.

22. Tan E, Levell N, Garioch J. The effect of a dermatology restricted-referral list upon the volume of referrals. Clin Exp Dermatol 2007;32(1):114–5.

23. Atwan A, Piguet V, Finlay AY, et al. Dermatology Life Quality Index (DLQI) as a psoriasis referral triage tool. Br J Dermatol 2017;177(4):e136–7.

24. Parthasarathy V, Pollock JR, McNeely GL, et al. A cross-sectional analysis of trends in dermatology practice size in the United States from 2012 to 2020. Arch Dermatol Res 2022. https://doi.org/10.1007/s00403-022-02344-0.

25. Record Number of Health-Care Deals Close 2021 With a Bang. 2022.

26. Nikpay SS, Richards MR, Penson D. Hospital-Physician Consolidation Accelerated In The Past Decade In Cardiology, Oncology. Health Aff 2018;37(7): 1123–7. https://doi.org/10.1377/hlthaff.2017.1520.

27. Berman B. Referral marketing: Harnessing the power of your customers. Bus Horiz 2016;59(1):19–28.

28. Szeto MD, Mamo A, Afrin A, et al. Social Media in Dermatology and an Overview of Popular Social Media Platforms. Current Dermatology Reports 2021;1–8.

29. Sivesind TE, Najmi M, Oganesyan A, et al. Social Media for Marketing and Business Promotion in Dermatology. Current Dermatology Reports 2021;1–8.

30. Ross NA, Todd Q, Saedi N. Patient seeking behaviors and online personas: social media's role in cosmetic dermatology. Dermatol Surg 2015;41(2): 269–76.

31. Albeshri M, Altalhab S, Alluhayyan OB, et al. The influence of modern social media on dermatologist selection by patients. Cureus 2020;12(12):e11822.

32. McLawhorn AS, De Martino I, Fehring KA, et al. Social media and your practice: navigating the surgeon-patient relationship. Current reviews in musculoskeletal medicine 2016;9(4):487–95.

33. Modahl M, Tompsett L, Moorhead T. Doctors, patients & social media. Quantia, MD: CareContinuum Alliance; 2011.

34. Loh CH, Tam SYC, Oh CC. Teledermatology in the COVID-19 pandemic: a systematic review. JAAD international 2021;5:54–64.

35. Vyas KS, Hambrick HR, Shakir A, et al. A systematic review of the use of telemedicine in plastic and reconstructive surgery and dermatology. Ann Plast Surg 2017;78(6):736–68.

# Asset Protection for Dermatologists
## An Overview on Shielding Wealth from Potential Liability

David B. Mandell, JD, MBA[a,b,*], Carole C. Foos, CPA[b],
Jason M. O'Dell, MS, CWM[b]

**KEYWORDS**

- Asset protection • Liability • Lawsuits • Exemption • Limited liability companies • Trusts

**KEY POINTS**

- Dermatologists face a host of potential legal risks both at the practice and through personal activities.
- Asset protection is a wealth planning discipline aimed at shielding a client's assets from potential future liability.
- Many dermatologists are misinformed as to their present risk exposure due to commonly believed asset protection myths.
- Asset protection tools can be plotted along a sliding scale of efficacy.
- Exempt assets, co-ownership forms, and legal tools all play a role in asset protection planning and have their pros and cons.

The reality of dermatology practice in the 21st century includes the potential for lawsuits and liability. While medical malpractice may be top-of-mind, there are a host of liability risks beyond malpractice–from employee claims and fiduciary liability for the practice retirement plan to premises liability and HIPAA violations– as well as potential personal liability for rental properties, car accidents (for self and children), outside businesses, personal guarantees and more.

In this article, we will outline the leading tactics and strategies dermatologists can utilize to better shield their assets from all sources of potential liability. Before we do so, we should first dispel some common misconceptions many dermatologists may have.

## COMMON MISCONCEPTIONS REGARDING ASSET PROTECTION
### "My Assets Are Owned Jointly with My Spouse, or by My Spouse Alone, so I'm Okay"

Most married dermatologists hold their homes and other property in joint ownership. Unfortunately, this ownership structure provides little asset protection in most states.

In community property states, community assets will be exposed to community debts regardless of title. Community debts include any debt that arises during marriage as the result of an act that helped the community. Certainly, any claims resulting from a medical practice, income-producing asset (rental real estate), or auto accident would be included.

[a] OJM Group, LLC, 401 East Las Olas Boulevard, Suite 1400, Fort Lauderdale, FL 33301, USA; [b] OJM Group, LLC, 8044 Montgomery Road, Suite 440, Cincinnati, OH 45236, USA
* Corresponding author. 401 East Las Olas Boulevard, Suite 1400, Fort Lauderdale, FL 33301.
*E-mail address:* mandell@ojmgroup.com

0733-8635/23/© 2023 Elsevier Inc. All rights reserved.

derm.theclinics.com

Even in non-community property states, joint property is typically at least 50% vulnerable to the claims against either spouse. Therefore, in most states, at least 50% of such property will be vulnerable—and all of the other problems associated with joint property still exist in non-community property states. The exception here is in states that have tenancy by the entirety (TBE), which we discuss later in the article.

Having the non-vulnerable spouse own title to the couple's assets does not protect the asset in most states. The creditor is often able to seize assets owned by the spouse of the debtor by proving that the income or funds of the debtor spouse were used to purchase the asset. To determine if the asset is reversible, 3 questions can be asked.

- Whose income was used to purchase the asset?
- Has the vulnerable spouse used the asset at any time?
- Does this spouse have any control over the asset?

If the answer is "yes" to any of these questions, then the creditor may be able to reach these assets.

### "I Am Insured, So I'm Totally Covered"

While we strongly advocate insurance as a first line of defense, and a fundamental part of any asset protection plan, an insurance policy is 50 pages long for a reason. Within those numerous pages are a variety of exclusions and limitations that most people never take the time to read, let alone understand. Even if you do have insurance and the policy does cover the liability in question, there are still risks of underinsurance, strict liability, and bankruptcy of the insurance company. In any of these cases, you could be left with the sole financial responsibility for the loss. Lastly, with losses that fall within the plan's coverage limits, you still may see your future premiums go up significantly.

### "I Can Just Give Assets Away if I Get into Trouble"

Another common misconception regarding asset protection is that you can simply give away or transfer your assets if you ever get sued. If this were the case, you could just hide your assets when necessary. You wouldn't need an asset protection specialist. You would only need a shovel and some good map-making skills so you could find your buried treasure later.

Recognizing the possibility that people may attempt to give away their assets when facing liability, there are laws prohibiting fraudulent transfers (also called or fraudulent conveyances or "voidable transfers"). In a nutshell, if you make an asset transfer after an incident takes place (whether you knew about the pending lawsuit or not), the judge has the right to rule the transfer a fraudulent conveyance and order the asset to be returned to the transferor, thereby subjecting the assets to the claims of the creditor. The law can even allow such a result if the transfers were made before the incident of liability, if it were *reasonably foreseeable* (eg, making transfers knowing you may soon default on a loan, even though the default hasn't occurred yet).

If you have been sued or suspect that you may be sued, there may be significant limitations to protection. Typically, reactive last-minute strategies are not effective, may be much more expensive than the highly successful strategies that can be implemented when there is no reasonably foreseeable claim, and can even compound liability in the worst circumstances.

## THE SLIDING SCALE OF ASSET PROTECTION

The most common misconception among physicians regarding asset protection is the idea that an asset is either "protected" or "unprotected." This "black or white" analysis is no more accurate in the field of asset protection than it is in the field of medicine. In fact, asset protection advisors are very similar to physicians in how they approach a client or patient.

Like a dermatologist who judges the severity of a patient's illness, asset protection specialists use a rating system to determine the protection or vulnerability of a client's particular asset. The sliding scale runs from−5 (totally vulnerable) to +5 (superior protection). As you have probably already guessed, our goal is to bring a client's score closer to (+5) for each of their assets.

Note on **Fig. 1**: The scale's lowest and highest values are straightforward and agreed-upon by advisors in the field–assets owned in one's own name, where no exemption applies are totally vulnerable to claims (−5) – while state or federally exempt assets (described later in discussion) are totally shielded, as are irrevocable trust assets in the right circumstances, so long as fraudulent transfer laws are no implicated. Between the extremes of (−5) and (+5), the protection degree is more variable, as there may be significant variability in state law–where the same tool in state A is very protective and quite weak in state B. Further, in the middle of the scale, experts in the field may disagree on the exact protection level or which tool is best among options.

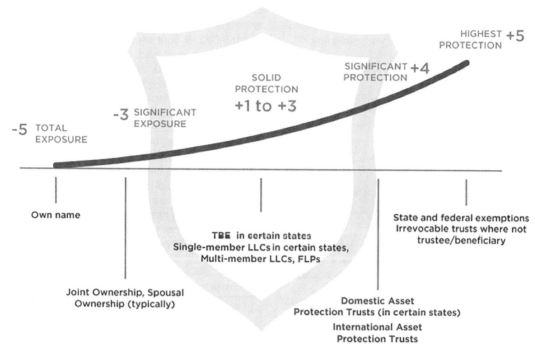

HIGHEST **+5**
PROTECTION

SIGNIFICANT **+4**
PROTECTION

SOLID
PROTECTION
**+1 to +3**

**-3** SIGNIFICANT
EXPOSURE

**-5** TOTAL
EXPOSURE

Own name

State and federal exemptions
Irrevocable trusts where not
trustee/beneficiary

TBE in certain states
Single-member LLCs in certain states,
Multi-member LLCs, FLPs

Joint Ownership, Spousal
Ownership (typically)

Domestic Asset
Protection Trusts (in certain states)

International Asset
Protection Trusts

**Fig. 1.** Asset protection sliding scale. *The scale presumes tools are created and utilized properly and when fraudulent transfer rules will not apply.

## EXEMPT ASSETS: THE "BEST" ASSET PROTECTION TOOLS

We consider exempt assets to be the best asset protection tool for the following reasons.

### No Legal/Accounting Fees

Most of the tools in subsequent articles involve the creation of legal entities that require set up and ongoing legal fees, state fees, accounting fees, and even additional taxes. Using the exempt assets described in this article involve none of these significant costs and affords better protection as well.

### No Loss of Ownership or Control

The legal tools of the following articles typically require giving up some level of ownership or control to family members or even third-party trustees. By using exempt assets, you can own and access the asset at any time while enjoying the highest (+5) level of protection.

### Superior Protection

The legal tools explained later offer protection that ranges from (+1) to (+5). Exempt assets always enjoy the top (+5) protection up to their exempt amount.

## FEDERALLY EXEMPT ASSETS

Federally exempt assets are those assets that are protected under federal bankruptcy law. Federal law protects certain assets from creditors and lawsuits if the defendant is willing to file bankruptcy to eliminate the creditor. In a Chapter 7 Bankruptcy, the debtor will be able to keep any assets that federal law deems exempt. The 2 significant asset classes that federal law protects are qualified retirement plans (QRPs) and IRAs. The term "qualified" retirement plan means that the retirement plan complies with certain Department of Labor and Internal Revenue Service rules. For the protection to apply, the plan should also comply with the Employee Retirement Income Security Act (ERISA). Most plans with non-owner employees will, but be sure to check on your plan.

You might know QRPs by their specific type, including profit-sharing plans, money purchase plans, 401(k)s or 403(b)s. IRAs are very similar to these plans with several technical differences, and are now given exempt status under the federal law as well.

While this protection is (+5), you must recognize that this federal protection only applies if you are in a bankruptcy setting and have access to the federal exemptions.

If you do not file for bankruptcy, this federal protection would not apply. The amount of value in the

QRP or IRA that would be protected outside of bankruptcy, like an ordinary lawsuit and creditor action, would be governed by your state law.

## STATE EXEMPT ASSETS

State exemption leveraging is a fundamental part of a financial plan and one which every doctor should take seriously. The most significant state exemptions are.

1. Qualified Retirement Plans and Individual Retirement Accounts
2. Primary Residence (or Homestead)
3. Life Insurance
4. Annuities

Important Note: We will make general comments regarding state exemptions later in discussion. These are NOT meant to be entirely accurate for any particular state.

### Qualified Retirement Plans and Individual Retirement Accounts

Most, but not all, states have significant (+5) exemptions for qualified retirements plans and IRAs. Some states protect only a certain amount in such asset classes or protect qualified plans more significantly than they do IRAs. It is crucial that a dermatologist understand the exemptions for these assets in their state and build their wealth accordingly.

### Primary Residence: Homestead

Many physicians consider the home to be the family's most valuable asset. You may have thought you knew the laws that protect your home. Perhaps you have previously heard the term *homestead*, and assumed that you could never lose your home to bad debts or other liabilities because of this homestead protection. The reality is that few states provide a total (+5) shield for the home.

Most states only protect between $10,000 and $60,000 of the homestead's equity. Some states, such as New Jersey, has no homestead protection statute, while other states, such as Florida[1] provide unlimited protection (with some restrictions). Consider today's real estate values and the equity that many doctors have in their homes, and it becomes clear that most states' homestead exemptions provide inadequate protection.

To determine how well a homestead law protects your home, you should compare the protected value to the equity. In order to do so, subtract the value of any mortgages from the fair market value of your home. For example, if you live in a home with a $300,000 fair market value and have a $150,000 mortgage, then your equity is $150,000. If your state protects only $20,000 through its homestead law, then you still have $130,000 ($150,000 of equity—$20,000 homestead) of vulnerable equity.

Homestead protection is often automatic, but may require additional action in some cases. Each state has specific requirements for claiming homestead status. In some states, you must file a declaration of homestead in a public office. Other states set a time requirement for residency before homestead protection is granted. Never assume your home is protected. You may be wrong and your inaction may cost you the protection you deserve. Your asset protection advisor can show you how to comply with the formalities in your state.

### Life Insurance

All 50 states have laws that protect varying amounts of life insurance. For example,.

- Many states shield the entire policy proceeds from the creditors of the policyholder. Some also protect against the beneficiary's creditors.
- States that do not protect the entire policy proceeds set amounts above which the creditor can take proceeds.
- Many states protect the policy proceeds only if the policy beneficiaries are the policyholder's spouse, children, or other dependents.
- Some states protect a policy's cash surrender value in addition to the policy proceeds. This can be the most valuable exemption opportunity.

### Annuities: Shielded in many States

An annuity is another exempt asset in many states. Annuities are insurance contracts that offer the upside of investment appreciation, tax-deferred growth, and principal protection. This diverse list of benefits makes annuities important components of asset protection and wealth accumulation plans.

### Quasi-Exemption: Tenancy by the Entirety

Tenancy by the Entirety ("TBE") is not a (+5) exempt asset, but it is a state law-controlled form of joint ownership that can provide total protection against claims against one spouse. TBE is available in about 20 states, although its effectiveness is diminishing. In some of these states, TBE only protects real estate; in some states both real estate and personal property (like bank accounts) can be effectively shielded by TBE. In those states that protect it, assets held in TBE cannot be taken by a party with a claim against only one spouse. These assets are immune to such a claim.

While this is a very powerful benefit, there are some risks with TBE, including.

### a. Joint Claim Risk

TBE provides no shield whatsoever against joint risks, including lawsuits that arise from your jointly owned real estate or acts of minor children.

### b. Divorce Risk

If you rely on TBE for protection and you get divorced before or during the lawsuit, you lose all protections from TBE.

### c. Survivor Risk

If you rely on TBE for protection and one spouse dies before or during the lawsuit, you lose all protections from TBE.

## LIMITED LIABILITY COMPANIES: THE BUILDING BLOCKS OF ASSET PROTECTION

While (+5) exempt assets may be the most effective asset protection tools, most dermatologists will need to go beyond the use of exempt assets in their quest to protect assets, and will make use of legal tools as well. Of all the legal tools used to shield assets, the most popular are limited liability companies (LLCs).

## HOW LIMITED LIABILITY COMPANIES PROTECT ASSETS?

In order to understand how LLCs provide protection, we must first examine both *inside risks* and *outside risks*. Inside risks are those which threaten the business and its assets because of the activity of the business. Examples of inside risks would be lawsuits against the business by its customers for product liability, by its patients for malpractice, or by its employees for wrongful termination. The LLC cannot shield the business itself from such inside claims. The only way to protect the business from inside claims is to protect the assets and cash flow of the business from potential business creditors. At minimum, protection can be achieved through proper insurance coverages, as noted earlier in the article.

We just wrote that "the LLC cannot shield the business itself from such inside claims," but what about the owners of the business? For example, if there is claim against the business for product liability, are the business owners' assets vulnerable?

In the LLC, none of the members are liable for the debts of the business.

Outside risks are potential claims against the owner(s)' interests in the business itself. For example, an outside claim might be a successful car accident lawsuit against the owner of the business where the plaintiff now wants to get to the assets of the business to satisfy the judgment. For outside risks, LLCs are asset protectors because the law gives a very specific and limited remedy to creditors coming after assets in this type of entity. When a personal creditor pursues you and your assets are owned by an LLC, the creditor cannot seize the assets in the LLC. Under the Uniform Act provisions, a creditor of an LLC member cannot reach into the LLC and take specific partnership assets.

If the creditor cannot seize LLC assets, what can the creditor get? The law normally allows for only one remedy: the charging order, which is something a creditor can be granted by a court against a debtor's interest in an LLC. Essentially, this order allows the creditor to get distributions.

In other words, the creditor must legally be paid any distributions that would have been paid to the debtor. The charging order is meant to allow the entity to continue operating without interruption and provide a remedy for creditors to be paid. However, as you will see, the charging order is generally a very weak remedy.

Of course, this discussion assumes that, in transferring assets to an LLC, you do not run afoul of fraudulent transfer laws. We introduced the concept of these laws earlier in this article. It also assumes that one remains in compliance with state laws and does not use the LLC as an alter ego of one's personal affairs.

## THE LIMITATIONS OF THE CHARGING ORDER

As mentioned earlier, the charging order is a court order which instructs the LLC to pay the debtor's share of distributions to his/her creditor until the creditor's judgment is paid in full. More importantly, everything we will describe later in discussion assumes that your LLC operating agreement is properly drafted and all formalities are followed. If these are handled, the charging order neither.

- Gives the creditor LLC voting rights
- Gives the creditor LLC management rights
- Forces the LLC manager to pay out any distributions to members

While the charging order may seem like a powerful remedy, one should consider its limitations. It is a temporary interest that may have to be renewed. In addition.

### It Is only Available After a Successful Lawsuit

First, the charging order is only available after the creditor has successfully sued you and won a judgment. Only then can your creditor ask the court for the charging order.

### It Does Not Afford Voting Rights—So You Stay in Control

Despite the charging order, you remain the managing member/manager of the LLC. You make all decisions about whether the LLC buys assets, distributes earnings to its partners or members, shifts ownership interests and so forth. Judgment creditors cannot vote you out because they cannot vote your shares. Thus, even after creditors have a judgment against you, you still make all decisions concerning the LLC, including whether to pay distributions to the owners.

### The Creditor May Have to Pay the Tax Bill

One element of advanced LLC planning is how the charging order may backfire on creditors for income tax purposes. Because taxes on LLC income are passed through to the parties who are entitled to the income, the LLC does not pay tax. Each partner/member is responsible for his/her share of the LLC income. This income is taxable regardless of whether the income is actually paid out.

If a creditor with a charging order against an LLC member goes to the step of *foreclosing* on the charging order, the creditor's interest will then become permanent. With the proper provisions in the LLC operating agreement, this may have the effect of making the creditor liable for all of the income attributable to the charged interest. At this point, the creditor "steps into your shoes" for income tax purposes with respect to the LLC interest—resulting in the receipt of your tax bill for income taxes on your share of the LLC income. This tax liability will exist even though the creditor will likely never receive any income. Once this occurs, creditors will be very motivated to settle, as they have swallowed the tax "poison pill" without even realizing it.

### PRACTICAL TIP: IF POSSIBLE, USE LIMITED LIABILITY COMPANIES IN THE MOST PROTECTIVE STATES

Not all LLCs are created equal. It is true that LLCs vary greatly in their asset protection, estate, and tax benefits based on the experience and expertise of the attorneys drafting the operating agreements. However, the point here is that some states have much more protective language in their LLC statutes than other states.

For some assets, like investment accounts, you may have the option to use LLCs in more protective states than your own. Some states, such as Nevada and Ohio, have passed extremely restrictive LLC statutes designed to provide the highest level of protection for entities established in their state.

Today, many doctors use an investment firm based outside of their state of residence, such as OJM Group, LLC, which manages investments for physicians in 48 states. Additionally, many physicians' assets managed by these firms are actually held by large custodians (such as Schwab or TD Ameritrade) in a third state. This type of asset, as opposed to real estate which always sits in one fixed place, may be suitable for ownership in an LLC outside of your home state. This type of "jurisdiction shopping" is found in numerous areas of the law, including estate planning, tax planning, and regulatory planning.

For example, you might live in your home state and set up an LLC in Ohio for its top-level protection laws. Your litigation risk still resides in your home state, where you live and practice medicine. Certainly, if you were ever sued, it would likely be in your home state and, if your LLC were attacked by a plaintiff in your home state, a court overseeing that lawsuit may be inclined to apply local law even when looking at an Ohio LLC. Nonetheless, if the costs of using a "better LLC state" like Ohio is not much more than setting up an LLC in your home state (or even less), then we generally recommend it; you can save costs and perhaps avail yourself of better protection rules. In essence, if it doesn't cost you a lot more to use a more protective state, there is really no reason not to so do.

Ideally, dermatologists will use legal entities domiciled in jurisdictions that offer the most favorable laws and make sure that a member of their advisory team is an asset protection expert, who will monitor developments in the field so that they can switch state domiciles if necessary.

### PRACTICAL TIP: BEWARE OF SINGLE-MEMBER LIMITED LIABILITY COMPANIES

The origin of charging order protections goes back to partnership law where the policy goal was to keep the business activities of a partnership from being disrupted by the non-partnership-related debts of individual partners. The concept underlying this policy was that interrupting the partnership business to satisfy the claim against one liable partner for a debt unrelated to the partnership was judged to be unfair to the innocent partners.

This origin now applies to LLCs. However, what about a single owner LLC? If you own 100% of an LLC and then have creditor issues, why shouldn't that creditor be able to penetrate the LLC, as there are no innocent LLC members who would be harmed?

This exact question has been raised by plaintiffs when attacking single-member LLCs, and it has been successful in a number of high-profile asset protection cases, including the *Olmstead* case[2] in Florida and the *Albright* case[3] in Colorado. These courts allowed penetration into single-member LLCs essentially because they had no other innocent owners. In response to these cases, several state legislatures amended their LLC statutes to specifically prevent this from happening against single-member LLCs in their states.

What does this mean for dermatologists who are single? At minimum, it means that they should form LLCs, when feasible, in states where the statutes specifically forbid such treatment of single-member LLCs. However, even married physicians should be concerned when using LLCs (or living) in states where single-member LLCs appear to be vulnerable. A court might view an LLC owned 100% by a married couple as, in substance, a single-member LLC. Perhaps this risk is even more pronounced in community property states like many of those in the West.

The bottom line: Unless you live in a state with a clear single-member LLC protective statute and are using an LLC in such a state, it makes sense to discuss with your asset protection advisor the value of an ongoing gifting program of LLC interests to children or other family members. The farther you are from a single-member LLC in form and in substance, the better position your entity will be against outside claims.

## USING TRUSTS TO SHIELD WEALTH

In addition to exempt assets and LLCs, a trust is another tool that can be used to protect dermatologists' assets and maintain their wealth. There are two categories of trusts: *revocable trusts* and *irrevocable trusts*. While revocable trusts (such as "family" or "living" trusts) can be quite valuable when it comes to estate planning, because they can be revoked/amended, they provide no asset protection while you (as the *grantor* or person who formed the trust) is alive.

## IRREVOCABLE TRUSTS: THE ASSET PROTECTORS

While revocable trusts offer no asset protection, irrevocable trusts are outstanding for asset protection. Of course, this discussion assumes that in transferring assets to any irrevocable trust, you

do not run afoul of fraudulent transfer laws, as discussed at the outset of this article.

While there are many types of irrevocable trusts, most have estate planning as their primary focus, even though they protect assets from liability as well. For brevity here, we will discuss the one irrevocable trust that is focused specifically on shielding assets from potential lawsuits.

## DOMESTIC ASSET PROTECTION TRUSTS

DAPTs are unique irrevocable trusts in that you can be both the grantor (the person establishing the trust) and a beneficiary of the trust–one who has access to trust assets. When there is no lawsuit concern, you can get to the trust assets as beneficiary. But if you have lawsuit claimants after you, the trust can be written so that the trustee cannot make distributions to you, as you are "under duress." In this way, a DAPT can allow you both access to the trust assets when the coast is clear and protection when lawsuits and creditors are at bay. As such, it can be very attractive for dermatologists who live and practice in a state with DAPT trust legislation. In these states, we would generally consider a DAPT to be at least a (+4) type of tool, and a (+5) tool in states where the DAPT law has been in place for some years because state law enshrines these protections.

Dermatologists in non-DAPT states may be able to take advantage of a DAPT in a foreign state if the trust is drafted in a way that complies with their home state law (this is called a "hybrid" DAPT or HDAPT). This strategy may involve attorneys in the DAPT state, as well as in the physician's home state, working together.

## SUMMARY

The reality of dermatology practice in the 21st century includes the potential for lawsuits and liability. This article outlines the leading tools dermatologists can utilize to better shield their assets from potential liability. The authors welcome your questions.

## DISCLOSURE

"None of the authors have any relevant relationships with firms that provide healthcare goods and services."

## REFERENCES

1. Florida Constitution Article X, Section 4.
2. Olmstead v. FTC - 44 So. 3d 76 (Fla. 2010).
3. In re Albright, 291 B.R. 538 (Bankr. D. Colo. 2003).

# Building a Group Practice and Going Big

David M. Pariser, MD,

## KEYWORDS

• Private practice group • Growing practice • Practice expansion

## KEY POINTS

- Growing a private practice is one way to remain independent in the changing health care environment.
- A large practice has advantages in the marketplace such as the ability to offer full service in dermatology to the public.
- Large practices can afford professional management, sophisticated electronic record keeping, and in-house information technology support and may be able to negotiate with payers.

In 1946, a young dermatologist who trained in dermatology at the University of Pennsylvania completed wartime service in the US Public Health Service and settled in the gritty Navy town of Norfolk, Virginia. There was only one physician practicing as a dermatologist within a 3+ hour drive and he was not formally trained. The "new kid in town," my father, Harry Pariser, was able to combine his fledgling private practice of dermatology with his real interest, the treatment of syphilis and other "venereal diseases." Training in sexually transmitted diseases, particularly syphilis defined the early practice of dermatology and was a major part of classical training in dermatology and syphilology in the 1930s.[1] The Norfolk, Virginia, Public Health Department was glad to have such an expert to run its "VD Clinic" which he did until the late 1970s.

I joined that practice in 1976 and my brother joined 2 years later. Fast forward to 2023, we are now an independent private practice with 21 board-certified dermatologists, 7 physician assistants (PAs), and one nurse practitioner (NP) with 7 locations in eastern Virginia. We have fellowship-trained Mohs surgeons, a full dermatopathology laboratory with fellowship-trained dermatopathologists, and a very active clinical research unit. In 2022, we treated over 130,000 patients in the clinical practice even in the face of the COVID pandemic. I have also been the principal investigator in over 600 clinical trials. We are closely associated with the Eastern Virginia Medical School's Department of Dermatology. We continue to maintain a close, but independent, relationship including the funding of a dermatology resident who rotates through our practice.

How did all that happen? I think it was a combination of factors: a sense of the need in the area, the demographics of the area, and the medical community; an awareness of what was going on in dermatology on a state and national level; the ability to change with the times; taking advantage of opportunities as they arose; the desire to be a "full-service" dermatology practice; the ability to recruit and retain qualified dermatologists and other clinicians; not being afraid to try new ideas and adopt new procedures; general knowledge about how to run a business; and most of all an entrepreneurial spirit. A guiding principle above all was and continues to be the delivery of the best possible dermatologic care to patients in the community regardless of demographic.

The advice that I am giving in this article represents lessons earned over 50 years of being a

Private Practice, Department of Dermatology, Eastern Virginia Medical School, 6160 Kempsville Circle Suite 200A, Norfolk, VA 23502, USA
*E-mail address:* dpariser@pariserderm.com

Dermatol Clin 41 (2023) 635–641
https://doi.org/10.1016/j.det.2023.05.002

dermatologist and having guided the expansion of a solo practice to a multi-provider unified full-service independent group.

## ADVANTAGES OF A BIG DERMATOLOGY PRACTICE

- *You can offer "Full Service."* This means that you can provide medical, surgical, esthetic, and other clinical services as well as dermatopathology. It may also mean that you may have more than one location. This in turn means that you will need more provider(s). Having multiple locations in the geographic area can be an advantage when dealing with payers as a larger demographic of patients can be served. Just because you are offering "full service" does not mean that you could not have specialized services and providers with specialized expertise such as contact dermatitis, complex medical dermatology, cutaneous oncology, and so forth. Being "full service" can also mean that you will be better able to serve the general population and will be able to accept patients without regard to insurance coverage as the efficiencies of a large practice will make up for lower reimbursement from some payers. "Full service" also means that there will be a mix of revenue sources including insurance reimbursement and cash-pay services

- *You can afford professional management.* If you started out as a small "Mom and Pop" practice and did most of the management yourself, you will find that it is not efficient for you to continue to manage it yourself as the job becomes larger.[2] You need help with hiring and firing, employee scheduling, benefit design, purchasing of equipment and supplies, negotiations with payers, leases and contracts, paying bills and collecting payments from patients and insurers, and numerous other day-to-day activities and problems that may become the source of frustration and burn out. It is not always the best idea to have the management done by an employee who may have been with you for a long time but who does not have management skills or prior management experience. Sometimes a very good Indian does not make a good Chief. You do not need an advanced degree but be on the lookout for someone who has managed a smaller medical practice in your community (preferably dermatology, but not necessarily) and is looking for more of a challenge.

- In addition to your practice administrator, it is essential as you grow to have high-quality support staff such as a financial officer who can be responsible for the big picture and can work with the practice outside accountants to take advantage of time-sensitive tax benefits as well as keeping track of financial trends. Also important is maintaining a relationship with an attorney knowledgeable in health care to assist in various aspects of the practice's business such as employment contracts, payer negotiations, and merger discussions if such an opportunity arises. Also critical is one or more employees, depending on need, who are experts in billing and coding for dermatology as well as employee(s) who deal with the ever-changing but constantly frustrating task of obtaining pre-authorization for medications and procedures. You spend the time with the patients. It is important that you properly bill and code for the procedures that you perform to get paid properly. Your billing and coding manager should be certified by the American Association of Professional Coders. As you grow it may become profitable as well as convenient to have in-house information technology support. Support for your coding questions is available from the American Academy of Dermatology.[3]

- *You don't need to skimp on space and support staff.* Payroll will likely be your largest expense but having well-trained support staff such as nurses and/or medical assistants will dramatically contribute to your efficiency in seeing patients, your productivity, and your quality of life in the practice. See what works best for all of your providers in terms of space and support staff. The degree of space and number of support staff may not be the same for all providers depending on their productivity. The efficient use of support staff is discussed later in this article.

- *You can afford a sophisticated electronic health record system.* In today's world of practice, proper documentation in the medical record is critically important not only to provide health care for patients but also to document services that were performed to justify billing and to have a complete record if any medico-legal problems arise. There are many electronic record systems on the market, some more friendly to dermatology than others. Qualified staff can help evaluate to see which perform best with the workflow of your practice. This is a critical decision so all should be involved.

- *You will have the ability to interact with colleagues.* As you will likely be practicing in the same location with others, you have the opportunity to have "instant" consultations and discussions about individual patients with your associates in real time.
- *You may have some negotiating leverage with payers.* Depending on the local payer mix in your area, your share of the dermatology market and the competitiveness of the payers, if you can offer full service in multiple locations you might have some leverage in negotiations.

## DISADVANTAGES OF GOING BIG

- *Acquiring and maintaining facilities.* Depending on the location, there may be some advantages as well as disadvantages to ownership of office space. Leasing space may be better if there is no ownership available in the desired location or access to capital is limited. When exploring a potential new location an important factor to consider is the presence of other competing dermatology practices in the area.
- If you are going to purchase or build the condominium or freestanding building, consider the purchase price, the cost of construction or renovations that you will need, the debt structure needed for financing, what will be needed for furnishing and equipping the office as well as the ongoing operating costs including insurance. A disadvantage of ownership is that it often means that you are wedded to that size of office in that location because it may be difficult to sell or lease the property if you outgrow the space or if you decide that there is a better location. If you are going to purchase a building or office condominium, it is a good idea to form a Limited Liability Company for each location.[4]
- For a rental, in addition to the monthly rent and annual escalation, what improvements will the landlord make to entice you to sign a lease, how much above and beyond the landlord's contribution will you need to pay for the renovations. Are real estate taxes, utilities, janitorial services, and insurance included are will you be charged separately?
- Be sure that the size of any proposed office space will be adequate not only for the immediate need but for foreseeable expansion during the term of the lease. Developing a relationship with a realtor and a space planner can be very helpful as they will have an idea of how much and what type of space and layout you need and can be a help in evaluating proposed now office locations.
- *People.* Probably the single biggest headache of managing a practice of any size revolves around people. Hiring and firing are an obvious task but management and retention of workers can be a challenge. It is important to develop a culture of inclusiveness and to let staff know that they are appreciated and that their opinions matter and suggestions that they make or problems that they identify are considered by management. Employee recognition programs which reward current performance and length of employment are helpful but personal recognition of the staff by the doctors goes a long way toward staff job satisfaction.
- Having a professional human resources manager to help with employment issues can not only help develop staff salary structures, can give advice on benefit structure including retirement planning and can conduct training of new employees. They can help keep the practice out of trouble from possible violation of employment laws. It is not just the staff who may present management problems. Strong-willed doctors may have very different ideas about various issues and preventing strife and trying to reach consensus can be a challenge
- *Lack of collegiality among providers.* As the practice grows, particularly if there is physical distance between offices and providers do not see each other regularly, discordance can develop in both the clinical practice and personal collegiality. For a big practice to remain cohesive and not to fragment, there needs to be a mechanism to develop and maintain a unified culture which the providers value.[5] Frequent meetings of all providers either in a business or in a social setting are important. The best way to develop a cohesive culture is for the senior and managing dermatologists to act by example, to be fair and not to take one side versus another when problems arise. When a contentious problem arises, try to reach compromise and consensus.
- *Organizational structure.* As the practice grows, there should be a defined organizational structure and a process for decision-making. Many physicians have an entrepreneurial spirit and want to be "owners" of the practice. They want to have a say in the management of the practice and input into decisions about growth. Others are happy being "employees" leaving decisions to others. There should be a place

for both. Having several "Vice-Presidents" and developing committees such as finance, cosmetic, long-range planning, clinical affairs, and so forth can be a way to include more doctors in the management of the practice and can take advantage of the skill set of the dermatologists who serve. Consideration should be given to compensation for officer and committee work to the extent that these functions detract from a physician's time which could otherwise be financially productive by seeing patients. Also, there should be some succession planning so that there is a mechanism for replacement of senior physicians, especially the managing partner, on death or retirement.

- *You will not have everything your way.* Compromise will be essential and decisions big and small need to be made by what is the best for the practice as a whole, not any individual or group.
- *You will not be able to have a cash-only practice.* In today's often frustrating world of the practice of medicine dealing with insurance payers and other regulations, the allure of becoming a cash-only practice and not dealing at all with insurance payers can seem to be an attractive option. This type of practice is not practical in many areas and works better with smaller, even solo, "boutique" practices. In fact if you dig a little you will find that these "boutique" practices usually accept Medicare patients. If you have a well-diversified practice there will be some cash-only services, usually esthetic as well an insurance reimbursement. Esthetic procedures sound nice as they are outside the payment structure defined by Medicare and insurers but price competition on the street for cosmetic services by nurses, PAs, and even medical assistants is fierce. The costs of these products have pulled much of the profit for physicians out of the procedure. Patients often shop by price and do not realize the skills needed for a good result. They may drop in to see you after the low-cost bad filler or muscle-relaxing experiment.

## FACTORS TO CONSIDER IF YOU WANT TO GO BIG

- *Get to know the demographics of the area and the local medical community.* Can you determine the need for dermatologic services in your area? You could do formal needs assessment, but it is probably just as good to ask your friends and family if they are having trouble getting an appointment with a dermatologist. Ask about their level of satisfaction with the providers that they have seen. You can also enlist a secret shopper to call your competition and find out how long the wait is to see a provider, and find out if they will see a dermatologist or extender. Part of the assessment of the local environment is the situation with insurance networks and the payer mix in the area.
- In some competitive areas, it may be difficult to join networks and as a solo or small practice you do not have much leverage with payers. It may be helpful if you develop a niche of expertise such as psoriasis, contact dermatitis, complex medical dermatology, clinical research, and so forth. Other articles in this volume discuss what it takes to go solo and the basic legal considerations of starting and maintaining a practice.[6] Legal advice and help with business management are essential when starting a practice and especially as you grow. A decision that you will need to make early on is whether you are going to want to grow organically by hiring new providers and opening new locations or whether you want to acquire smaller existing practices. The sometimes extremely high valuations paid to some practices by private equity and venture capital groups may make acquisition of existing groups out of financial reach. Other, older physicians may just hand their practice over in exchange for management of their paper records. Another option for growth is to merge with another group.[7] There are many factors to consider in a merger such as valuation of practice assets and liabilities. Consider debts or payments that you may be inheriting, how to handle receivables, management of discordances in salaries of professional and support staff and most of all, blending what might be different cultural ethos of both practices, not to mention the structure of leadership in the newly combined entity.
- *Be aware of what is going on in dermatology on a state and national level.* The latest trends in the practice of dermatology may not be coming to your town just yet but it is very helpful to get to know what is going on in other places. Of course, there are always advances in medical, surgical, and esthetic dermatology and it is important to keep up but it is also important to know what is going on in the fields of legislative and regulatory decisions that would impact the practice of dermatology as well as the shifts in insurance reimbursement, workforce issues, as well as added

administrative burdens. The American Academy of Dermatology, the American Society for Dermatologic Surgery, your state medical or dermatology society or any of the dermatology subspecialty societies will keep you informed and is a good way to get continuing medical education and to interact with colleagues in other areas of the country. It is beneficial to see what problems and opportunities have arisen and how they have been handled. Abraham Lincoln is credited with the quote "The best way to predict the future is to create it." Anticipating problems and dealing with them proactively can save a lot of headache down the line. Having the foresight to implement new programs such as patient safety initiatives, dermatopathology laboratory, specialized dermatologic surgery, or development of an esthetic practice can be the ways to create the future.

- *Take advantage of opportunities as they arise.* It is great to have visions of what your practice could be but pragmatism must play a part. Are there dermatologists available to recruit? You could want to grow by hiring new dermatologists but the reality may be that it is very difficult to hire newly minted dermatologists, especially in some areas of the country. Physician recruiters may be helpful in finding candidates but fees can be expensive, costing up to $250,000 per hire.[8]
- Get involved in the local medical school dermatology residency program on a voluntary position. This gives you not only the academic stimulation of interaction with residents but also it allows you to get to know individual residents and allows them to get to know you. This development of a relationship with residents in training can be a source of potential recruits for your practice. There may be a program for education of PAs or NPs in your city. If there is one and if you see the value of these nonphysician clinicians in your practice, you could offer the opportunity for students in these programs to spend some time with you. A properly trained and supervised PA or NP can bring an added dimension to a busy dermatology practice. Another opportunity can be to recruit the dermatologist spouse of a physician in another specialty who is coming to your town. Wherever the source of new physicians or mid-level providers is sure to carefully vet them with references from their training program or previous employment.
- *Recruit and retain good dermatologists and other staff.* Any physician who comes from an accredited dermatology residency program and passes the American Board of Dermatology examination is going to have the medical knowledge to practice but they may not have the personality or the ethos that matches that of your practice. Developing a culture of inclusiveness and collegiality is important, and it may be difficult to judge with just an interview or two. At the very least have the potential candidate shadow in the practice for several days and observe them in a social situation, such as a reception or a dinner. When possible get references from their training program or previous employer if applicable. Unless you have a personal relationship from the person giving the reference however you might not get much useful information.
- A key to retention of physicians (and all staff for that matter) is to treat them fairly and to be sure that they know that they are being treated fairly and are valued. Fairness should encompass the workplace to include the use of supporting staff, assignment of space to practice, and working schedule, but most important is that there should be a fair and a uniform formula for compensating the dermatologists usually based on their productivity. There should be a provision for part-time as well as full-time work for the younger generation of dermatologists starting a family and for the older ones nearing retirement.
- Create a mechanism for including the dermatologists in the organizational structure of the practice. Most want some ability to have input into decisions not just about clinical matters and issues pertaining directly to them, but also about practice governance, growth, inclusion of new providers, addition of new office locations, and so forth. The establishment of committees to deal with these types of issues is a way to promote inclusion and collegiality. Realize the different levels of interest in decision-making among dermatologists and that everyone should be appreciated for the contributions that they can make to the practice.
- Most of these comments about physician recruitment and retention apply to PAs and NPs, but the retention of support staff is somewhat different. Assuming that your practice is paying market rates to your staff and providing market benefits probably the most important aspect of staff retention is that the staff member feels that they are valued and that their work is appreciated. Specific recognition programs may be helpful but it is the day-to-day relations of the dermatologists with the staff that is most important.

- *Make the most of your nonphysician care team.* All dermatologists have a care team, whether it is a solo practitioner with one medical assistant or a large group practice with physician assistant (PAs), nurse practitioner (NPs), registered nurse (RNs), licenced practical nurse (LPNs), medical assistants, estheticians, scribes, histotechnologists (for a Mohs laboratory or for a full dermatopathology laboratory processing permanent sections). As health care delivery changes and the workforce shortage of dermatologists increases the efficient use of a health care team will give an added dimension of care to a busy practice no matter what size. It will allow the dermatologist to do what he or she does best, give patients more "face time," better education and more "hand holding" and in well accepted by patients and payers.

### Physician Assistant/Nurse Practitioners

A properly trained and supervised PA or NP can bring an added dimension of patient care to the practice as well as an additional source of revenue. Anytime patient care is delegated to a nonphysician, and there is a potential effect on the quality of care that is delivered by the practice. PAs and NPs do not receive enough dermatology education and experience in PA school to practice independently. It is important that the practice invest the time and resources in educating the newly-trained PA or NP so that they will be able to work as an extension of the dermatologist. Investing in the continuing education of these providers is also important to maintain quality patient care. It is beyond the scope of this article to describe in detail the specifics of a training program for PAs and NPs.[9] The amount and type of training will vary according to the PA/NPs prior experience and their anticipated duties in the practice. Education and professional development of the PA/NPs should be encouraged but if that they bring new procedures or services to the practice be sure that you are well versed in their performance and management of complications. In addition to routine medical dermatology services, PA/NPs can be trained to perform procedures such as cryosurgery, minor excisions, electrodesiccation and curettage (ED&Cs), I&Ds, biopsies, steroid injections, and cosmetic services such as toxin and filler injections.

### Medical Assistants

Getting the most use of medical assistants is one of the best ways to increase efficiency and productivity of the practice. In additional to the usual duties of ushering patients through the office flow and gathering medical history, they can be an extra set of hands assisting in procedures and can collect specimens such as for Potassuim Hydroxide (KOH) or cultures. Depending on the size of the practice, medical assistants can "specialize" in administration of phototherapy (ultraviolet light - A [UVA], UVB, excimer laser, photodynamic therapy) according to protocols. In certain states, they can be trained to perform very minor procedures such as removal of skin tags and certain biopsies where no medical judgment is needed in their performance. Please check with your State Board of Medicine before initiating such a program. Medical assistants can also double as scribes.

### Scribes

Efficiency and productivity can almost always be enhanced by the use of a scribe. Medical assistants can be trained to scribe for you while you are in the treatment room. A well-trained scribe can prepare the office note, whereas you and the patient are in the room. The use of macros can greatly facilitate the process of having the chart note done or nearly done before you leave the treatment room. If the scribe needs some clarification they can ask you immediately after leaving the patient's room. Many of the electronic record systems will automatically assign current procedure terminology (CPT) billing codes to the encounter or the scribe can be trained to code the visit. You should always review not only the medical entries but also the billing for each visit. A scribe can also serve as a chaperone freeing up other medical assistants or nurses to have time to perform other functions. A scribe can be a good financial investment. As an example, if you see 30 patients per day and it takes you 3 minutes to prepare a chart note it would take an hour and a half each day just to do the charting. The revenue that you would generate by using that hour and a half to see more patients would greatly exceed the cost of the salary and benefits of the scribe. Every provider should have a dedicated scribe. If you do not want to take the time to fully train a scribe there are commercial services that can provide scribe services, and some may even have training in dermatology, but in order to get the best benefit from a scribe you will need to do some individual training and incorporate the scribe into your office workflow.

- *Do not grow too fast.* Each time you add a provider or open a new location there are bound to be stresses on the practice and often unforeseen problems may arise. At each step be sure that your infrastructure is prepared starting with the people who answer the phone and the "back-office" personnel such as the billing clerks and pre-authorization co-ordinators to the medical assistants and other clinical personnel. Be sure that you are appropriately "staffed up" for each expansion of office space. Be sure that your administrative staff can handle the needed support of new providers or a new office location.

Twenty things to do and not do if you want to *Build a Group Practice and Go Big*.

- Be sure that there is a demand in your area for dermatologic services and get to know where in your area there is a need for expansion of dermatologic services.
- Become a full-service practice offering medical, surgical, pediatric, and esthetic services as well as dermatopathology.
- For office location expansion, weigh the pros and cons of ownership versus rental.
- Engage the services of a trusted accountant and attorney when you contemplate a major expansion of people or locations.
- When expanding to a new location be sure that the space you purchase or rent will accommodate anticipated growth in the near future.
- Do due diligence on recruiting new dermatologists or mid-level providers.
- Take advantage of opportunities such as hiring graduating residents from the local medical school residency program or dermatologists that are coming to your town for family reasons.
- Hire competent, experienced administrative staff as your practice grows.
- Invest the time and effort in professional development of your staff.
- Consider providing retail skin care products to patients in an ethical manner.
- Train and properly supervise physician assistants and nurse practitioners.
- Do not skimp on office personnel or staff.
- Get the most from your medical assistants and/or nurses.
- Develop a staff recognition program.
- Be sure that compensation and benefits for all employees is in line with others in your geographic area.
- Provide a scribe for each provider.

- Develop a formal system of practice governance that can allow the dermatologists who show interest in management of the practice to have input.
- Develop a presence beyond your practice by participating in groups such as the American Academy of Dermatology, your state or local dermatologic society, or one of the many sub-specialty societies in dermatology.
- Develop a succession plan for your replacement on death or retirement.
- Do not grow too fast.

## DISCLOSURE

No conflicts of interest to disclose.

## REFERENCES

1. Chu MB, Tarbox M. The role of syphilis in the establishment of the specialty of dermatology. JAMA Dermatol 2013;149(4):426.
2. Shanafelt TD, Gorringe G, Menaker R, et al. Impact of organizational leadership on physician burnout and satisfaction. Mayo Clin Proc 2015;90(4):432–40.
3. American Academy of Dermatology Association. CODING RESOURCE CENTER. Available at: https://www.aad.org/member/practice/coding. Accessed Mar 29 2023.
4. Watts, R, Bottorff C. How To Start An LLC In 7 Steps (2023 Guide). Available at: https://www.forbes.com/advisor/business/how-to-set-up-an-llc-in-7-steps/. Accessed Mar 29 2023.
5. American Medical Association. How to create a vibrant culture in your private practice. Available at: https://www.ama-assn.org/practice-management/private-practices/how-create-vibrant-culture-your-private-practice. Accessed Mar 29 2023.
6. Freedman, M. How to Open a Private Medical Practice, Step by Step. Available at: https://www.businessnewsdaily.com/8910-opening-a-medical-practice.html. Accessed Mar 29 2023.
7. Ironmark. 7 BEST PRACTICES FOR MERGING YOUR MEDICAL PRACTICE. Available at: https://blog.ironmarkusa.com/best-practices-merging-medical-practice. Accessed Mar 29 2023.
8. Healthcare Recruitment Link. What Will it Cost to Recruit a Physician? Available at: https://healthrecruitlink.com/blog/what-will-it-cost-to-recruit-a-physician. Accessed Mar 29 2023.
9. MacNeil JS. Make Your Extender a Dermatologist Clone. Available at: https://www.mdedge.com/content/make-your-extender-dermatologist-clone. Accessed Mar 29 2023.

# Musings from a Bent Arrow
## The Road from Private Practice to Academics

Kishan H. Pandya, MD[a,1], Robert T. Brodell, MD[b,c],*

## KEYWORDS

- Private practice • Academic medicine • Career • Educator's portfolio • Professor • Niche • Culture

## KEY POINTS

- Although it is more common for dermatologists in academics to enter private practice, it is entirely possible to transition from private practice to academics with proper planning.
- To most effectively transition to an academic career from private practice, it is essential to have an experienced academic mentor.
- Maintaining a prospective academic portfolio/curriculum vitae is essential to properly document the information that will be analyzed by a promotions and tenure committee during the transition to academics.

In twenty-first century America, it is common for individuals to change jobs many times during their working life. In the field of medicine, individuals may begin their career in academic medicine and then pivot to the private sector but somewhat less common to work in private or group practice and make a late career move to academics.[1] There are many reasons for this, not the least of which is the difficulty of a senior clinician moving into academics at the bottom of the academic food chain as an instructor or assistant professor.[2]

This article explores the method one of us (RTB) used to transition from a successful 27-year career in a private practice to become Founding Chair of a Department of Dermatology at a major medical center. The most significant factor that permitted this to happen was not innate ability or intelligence but rather the engagement of an academic mentor who provided guidance every step along the way while in private practice to prepare for an academic career. In fact, the transition was amazingly smooth because academic dermatology is increasingly like private practice. In fact, academic salaries across the country are being driven by relative value units (RVUs)[3,4] efficiency in clinical practice is increasingly important because research funds are drying up or concentrated in a few research universities.[5,6] Thus, private practitioners have specific, valuable skills that can be harnessed in the academic setting.

## A STORY OF TRANSITION FROM PRIVATE PRACTICE TO ACADEMICS: LUCK AND SERENDIPITY

After graduating from the University of Rochester School of Medicine and Dentistry in 1979, Robert Brodell spent 2 years of Internal Medicine training at Strong Memorial Hospital in Rochester, New York while his wife Linda Brodell completed her medical school training. They both transitioned to Washington University in St Louis for 3 years of training in dermatology and ophthalmology (1 year of Internal Medicine and 3 years of ophthalmology), respectively. This left an additional year that Bob could have invested in a private practice

Funding Sources: None.
a Summa Health System, Akron, OH, USA; b Department of Pathology, University of Mississippi Medical Center, Jackson, MS, USA; c Department of Dermatology, University of Mississippi Medical Center, Jackson, MS, USA
1 Present address: 55 Arch Street, Suite 1B, Akron, OH 44304.
* Corresponding author. 2500 North State Street, Jackson, MS 39216.
E-mail address: rbrodell@umc.edu

Dermatol Clin 41 (2023) 643–652
https://doi.org/10.1016/j.det.2023.05.003

opportunity to save money for developing a private practice on returning home to Warren, Ohio. Strong advice from Bob's father led him to "take this amazing opportunity to learn more." Daniel J. Santa Cruz, MD was the director of dermatopathology at the time and he offered to accept Bob as his first fellow in exchange for help writing the Program Information Form (PIF) required by the Dermatology and Pathology Residency Review Committees. Writing this PIF proved to be incredibly important at the transition to academics because it gave Bob confidence in one of the skills required decades later during the transition to academic medicine.

In 1985, the Doctors Brodell established a private practice in Bob's hometown of Warren, Ohio, living in the building where they worked for the next 27 years. The practice also included an optical ship and an independent certified dermatopathology laboratory. David R. Bickers, MD visited Bob, Stephen E. Helms, MD another dermatologist with an existing practice in Warren, and Dale R. Pokorney, MD a residency-mate of Bob's who had recently established his practice in Sharon, Pennsylvania, just across the Ohio border. At this dinner meeting, he invited all 3, heretofore referred to as the "three amigos," to teach in rotating fashion covering a monthly Thursday afternoon residents' clinic in Cleveland, Ohio, 60 miles away. Each of the 3 would volunteer 4 times per year and become members of the clinical faculty at CWRU.[7] This meeting was critical because it allowed Bob to keep his hand in academics and because it established David Bickers as his primary mentor for the next 40 years.

At a memorable meeting in the next month over beer and snacks while watching a Cleveland Browns football game, Dr Bickers asked Bob where he planned to be in his career in 5, 10, 20, and 30 years. The response: Bob would like to serve the people of Warren, Ohio, where he grew up and where his family and friends lived but would like to end this career in academic medicine at a university. Dr Bickers took a methodical approach to thinking through a plan, which would have a chance at success but came with no guarantees.

First, Bob would need to have a niche that could serve as the basis for an academic career.[8] Dr Bickers suggested that Warren was too far from Cleveland for me to spend the time each week required to establish an academic career at the bench in one of their laboratories. The solution arrived on was critical to all future academic success. Bob would take clinical images of every single lesion that was biopsied. Since this tissue was processed and read in an onsite laboratory, the

clinical material would be available on which to build a career rooted in clinical-pathologic correlation. Then, Dr Bickers suggested finding medical students to provide the energy and enthusiasm to write up the most interesting cases.[9]

Second, Dr Bickers asked if Bob was passionate about anything in dermatology. The frustrated response revolved around the American Board of Dermatology (ABD) certifying examination, which had just been taken. The emphasis of the complaint rested on the heavy emphasis of the examination on basic science and clinically irrelevant factoids. Dr Bickers suggested writing "better" questions using my clinical images and photomicrographs for the ABD, which could be funneled through their question-writing committees.

Third, he stated unequivocally that it would be best if Bob could be a professor by the time he was ready to transition to an academic career. It would be very difficult for a 50 or 60-year-old dermatologist to enter academic medicine at the level of an instructor or assistant professor. He noted that it would be nearly impossible for Bob to be promoted to Professor in the Department of Dermatology at Case Western Reserve University because of their stringent requirements and suggested joining the faculty at Northeastern Ohio Universities College of Medicine (NEOUCOM) in nearby Rootstown, Ohio, which has since been renamed, Northeast Ohio Medical University (NEOMED). In this position, Bob would have a chance at promotion to Professor with a little grit and determination.

Fourth, Dr Bickers suggested that Bob teach at every opportunity that presented itself. To teach is to learn twice, and he noted that teaching is a learned skill that comes with practice.[10] These skills proved to be central to the eventual transition to an academic position.

The 3 amigos agreed to give a lecture to the dermatology residents over lunch before each of the clinics where they served as a preceptor. Ultimately, Bob joined the clinical faculty at the University of Rochester School of Medicine where he gave a lecture and supervised a resident clinic every month that had 5 Fridays (about 4 times per year).

Fifth, Dr Bickers instructed Bob to prospectively keep track of every possible academic contribution that could serve as the basis for promotion.[11,12] This included not only peer-reviewed publications but also the names of medical students that were mentored with corresponding dates, the students for whom Bob wrote letters of recommendation, and articles reviewed for dermatology and pathology journals using the number of the submission, not the titles or authors.

It also included every lecture performed with date, topic and audience, awards, and dates of promotion at NEOMED.

Finally, Dr Bickers told Bob that the basis for any academic career is taking care of each patient in my private practice the very best I could. If one's clinical work is not "top notch," nothing else will evolve in the areas of research or education.[13–21]

Soon after the Bickers meeting, Bob joined the NEOUCOM faculty where there were no paid faculty teaching the third and fourth year medical students.[7] All clinical faculty were volunteers who taught medical students in their private offices. Motivated to reach academic goals, Bob became Section Head of the Department of Dermatology within several years, a position held for more than 2 decades.

There were several things that happened during Bob's private practice years that prepared him for a future academic career. None of these academic successes was predicted or well planned. They just happened.

### Learning from my Northeast Ohio Medical University Medical Students

When Bob began having medical students serving their dermatology electives, he thought he was giving back to repay the many teachers who were instrumental in his career. It soon became obvious that students were engaged in a symbiotic relationship rather than a parasitic one![22–24] Students were helping in many ways because they engaged in team-based care with Bob and his staff. Recognizing that many of these students needed a publication to prepare themselves for the rigorous dermatology matching process, Bob began to find cases that would serve as grist for the publication mill[9] and then the passion of students began to drive more complex projects.[25] Students also began to contribute in unexpected ways.

One student, Ashish Bhatia, had been in the computer business before attending medical school. In 1998, he told Bob about incredible machines that could project images on a screen from small computers called "laptops." He supervised the conversion of 80 lectures that were composed of Kodachrome slides stored in round carousels. Several high school students who served as file clerks in the office completed this work within a month. Becoming an early adopter of this technology allowed word slides to be changed in software immediately before a lecture rather than the 1 week turn-around required when word slides were mailed away to be produced. This capability became important in the next section!

### Becoming President of the American Board of Dermatology

After several years of submitting questions to the ABD test-writing committees, an amazing thing happened! Dr Bickers proved to be correct...an inexhaustible supply of questions based on clinical images and corresponding histopathology was something the ABD valued. In fact, Bob only submitted about 20 questions per year but after 4 years, they asked him to join a medical dermatology test-writing committee. It was clear; the ABD agreed that the certifying examination could be improved with more content that mirrored clinical practice.

My first test-writing committee meeting in Chicago was intense. About 8 or 9 famous dermatologists sat in a small room each with a 2.5 foot pile of papers stacked in front of them that included 320 questions on one page and a supporting scientific article in case there were issues raised with the validity of the answer. Each of committee member wrote suggested changes to the question, and the committee chair and his administrator went through all these piles of paper to construct the final edited questions to be contributed to the bank that year.

The next year, Bob arrived at the test committee meeting with the Ashish Bhatia approved laptop and digital projector. From 2 PM until 2 AM he entered all 320 questions. The next day these questions were projected on a wall while the traditional Kodachrome was projected on a screen as per usual. Bob typed in suggested edits by committee members to each questions in real time. At the end of the meeting, the test questions were complete. The committee members thought Bob was a computer genius. The next thing he knew, Bob was elected to the ABD Board of Directors, in part, because of his meager computer skills and, in part, for another reason. The board wanted the input of a private practitioner as the Maintenance of Certification (MOC) program was being rolled out. After 10 years on the Board of Directors (BOD), Bob became president of the ABD.... something that he never considered would be possible.

### Learning Leadership Skills Through Volunteer Work with the American Cancer Society Relay for Life

Soon after Bob moved to Warren, Ohio, his mother told him that he was expected to do something for the community. Bob was busy with a new private practice, financial worries, and a growing family. It *really* did not seem that there was time to add community service to this mix. He decided to present an annual public lecture at the Warren library on skin cancer. After a few years, Bob came to know several volunteers and it was clear to him that the organization he was growing to feel passionate about needed more than one skin cancer lecture per year. Bob subsequently became involved with every known "failed" American Cancer Society fundraiser: ducks down the river; handsome hunk contests; jail and bail; an art show and sale; and several variations on the American Cancer Society (ACS) door-to-door crusade. With 20 to 40 volunteers working many hours, the most money everyone made was US$4000 to 6000. Bob thought that only by involving youth in ACS activities would the organization have a future. The answer was clear: 3 on 3 basketball tournaments! Bob attended a national conference that included a session on raising money through basketball tournaments. Although learning about the promise and pitfalls of basketball fundraisers, Bob attended a session on the ACS Relay For Life (RFL).

The ACS RFL was an almost magical event. Everyone at the session was dressed in purple and enthusiastic about the promise of walking or running on a track for 24 hours following a survivor's lap at the beginning.[26] After Bob returned home, the board approved an event 6 weeks later, which raised US$28,000. He was on to something. Bob devoted his lunch hour to recruiting RFL teams from businesses, physician offices, and community groups several times per week. During its peak year, the Trumbull County RFL raised more than US$1 million. The ACS became a cauldron of opportunities to develop leadership skills,[27,28] leading to becoming president of the Ohio Division of the ACS and the East Central Division before taking a position on the national Board of Directors and the BOD of the Cancer Action Network, which led to involvement with a committee that innovated Celebration on the Hill in 2006 where 10,000 ACS volunteers from every congressional district descended on Washington, DC, to urge Congress to invest in cancer research programs. In good measure to this event, the NIH budget doubled in the next 5 years.

The RFL was the most impactful experience of Bob's life, and it taught several lessons. Never give up. Passion and hard work can take one a long way. His position in the community at a physician engendered respect that could be used to reach goals. Participating with Bob's family was fun and led to a special kind of learning for his kids related to "walking the walk" and not just "talking the talk." Finally, getting involved can enrich one's life in ways that could never have

been predicted regarding family, new friends, and incredible activities.

## The Amazing Experience of Being Able to End my Career in Academics as a Chairperson

At the end of a long day of moving furniture and boxes during a visit to St Louis in June 2011, Bob's daughter Lindsey Brodell Dolohanty was moved into an apartment and ready to start her residency training at Washington University in St Louis. An email from a recruiter read: "Looking for a Chair at a Southern University." Bob asked Linda about the possibility of ending his career in academics. In the past, the question "Is it time?" was met with derision: too risky….to many tuitions for children's education…. it was simply too good in Warren! This time, however, perhaps thinking about our years of training in St Louis, the question "Is it time?" with a one-word answer: "Maybe!" Bob responded to the recruiter's email and typed the answer to his question: "Am I interested?": "Maybe." Amazingly, the recruiter lived and worked in St Louis, Missouri. Bob and Linda met him the next day for breakfast and about the time the omelets arrived, the recruiter announced the position was at the University of Mississippi Medical Center (UMMC) in Jackson! The recruiter detected the disappointment in our faces, quickly responding to it with 5 words that Bob subsequently repeated a thousand times: "It's not what you think!"

Linda and Bob visited UMMC, and it was *not* at all what they thought. It was a vibrant medical center with almost 10,000 employees and a US$1.5 billion budget, the only academic medical center in this largely rural state. Giants in medicine had done the first heart transplant and were national leaders in medical physiology research and teaching. Most importantly, the university needed someone with Bob's skill set! Someone to run and grow a clinical practice. Someone to teach. Someone to recruit faculty. Someone to help medical students write clinical research articles to help them gain admission to dermatology residency programs. Someone to apply for a residency training program where there had never been one in the past. They did not need Bob to apply to the National Institutes of Health for RO1 grants, a skill that was not in his toolbox.

After an interview trip and providing answers to what seemed like an interminable number of questions, an amazing thing happened. The dean of UMMC offered Bob a job! Of course, Bob called David Bickers who had been guiding him through the interview process. Dr Bickers wrote the 12 things that UMMC would need to do if Bob was

---

**Box 1**
**The 12 "Asks" suggested by David Bickers for a new chair[a]**

1. You will serve as Division Chief of the Division of Dermatology

2. The Dean of the School of Medicine will approve Departmental Status for Dermatology as soon as the Dermatology Residency Review Committee (RRC) approves a residency program for our institution.

3. Once departmental status is approved, you will serve as Chair of the Department of Dermatology subject to having satisfactory evaluations as Division Chief. A salary range was included here.

4. In addition to the current faculty members and already committed recruit, we will provide nationally competitive salary support for the following individuals: a contact dermatitis specialist, a pediatric dermatologist, a general dermatologist, and a research scientist.

5. Adequate administrative, educational, and faculty office space

6. Salary support for a divisional/departmental business administrator

7. Salary support for the program coordinator for the residency program once it is established

8. Salary support for an administrative assistant for faculty members with a ratio consistent with other departments

9. In addition to current off-site locations, clinic space on campus with appropriate equipment, sufficient examination rooms, a conference area, an adjacent Mohs suite, and adjacent pathology laboratory space for the department. We will do our best to size this space to include the 12 examination rooms and 3 Mohs surgery rooms subject to volume projections and space constraints of the location selected. This will all be done with your input and approval.

10. Appropriate level medical assistant and nursing support in the clinics consistent with national and UP staffing levels.

11. Salary support of 2 residents per year.

12. All resources devoted to the division of dermatology will be transferred to the department of dermatology when departmental status is approved.

13. Dermatopathology and Mohs surgery as well as all practice of dermatology approved within the scope of training outlined by the dermatology RRC and/or the ABD may be practiced by the division/department of dermatology subject to privileges being granted in the standard fashion by the hospital medical staff office.

14. A salary, recruitment incentive, and moving expenses were stated.

[a]All were agreed to by the University of Mississippi Medical Center and all promises were kept.

---

going to take the job (**Box 1**). All of the things on the list were designed to set Bob up for success and for Bob getting the opportunity of a lifetime, failure was not an option.

After working 1 year in the Department of Otolaryngology with 2 excellent dermatologists who were recruited to teach Ear, Nose, and Throat residents' cosmetic procedures and a young, medical dermatologist fresh out of training, the dermatology RRC approved UMMC for a residency training program and Bob became Chair of the Department of Dermatology. As of the 2021/22 academic year, the department had graduated 21 dermatology residents in a state that had never had a program. With 11 residents in their PGY2-4 years and 5 in their transitional Internal Medicine Internship, accounting for another 16 residents, a total of 37 residents were trained or in training. One dermatopathology resident was trained and

one was in training. Four Mohs Fellows were trained, and one was in training.

The faculty include a Mohs surgeon, Cosmetic Dermatologist, Pediatric Dermatologist, 2 patch test/contact dermatitis specialists, and 2 dermatopathologists, 4 medical dermatologists, and a hospitalist dermatologist were running the only rural academic office at a great distance from a medical center, a skin lymphoma clinic, psoriasis clinic, a cosmetic clinic, a Skin Cancer Center and several free clinics while offering store-and-forward teledermatology consultations to rural primary care physicians and a Dermatology Project ECHO to educate primary care physicians once a month over lunch. Three nurse practitioners work in the clinics in tandem with faculty. More than 55,000 patient visits per year, 5500 dermatopathology accessions, 350 patch tests, and thousands of cosmetic procedures are performed annually. In the decade that the department has been in existence the residents wrote 15 AAD questions of the week and the faculty and residents generated 39 poster presentations, dozens of presentations at regional and national venues, 228 peer-reviewed publications, 22 book chapters, and 2 books. Grants totaled over US$510,000.

The Department of Dermatology was the first department at UMMC to have more than one Registered Nurse (RN)/Licensed Practical Nurse (LPN)/Medical Assistant (MA) per physician to help manage the demands of high-volume patient care with the complexities of EPIC™ electronic health record, earlier authorizations, and the myriad of requirements inherent in a large medical center.[29,30] The department became a national leader in offering access to care in rural areas.[31–33] It also became a leader in the application of Project ECHO[34] and store and forward telehealth to train rural primary care physicians and help their patients with dermatology problems.[35–38] The textbook written by the UMMC team, *Dermatology in Rural Settings: Organizational, Clinical, and Socieoeconomic Perspectives* was given the honor of being placed in the Elsevier Foundation Sustainable Development Goals Series and is the "go to" book addressing the maldistribution of dermatologists and the many solutions that can affect this problem.[39] The University of Mississippi was also the first dermatology department in the country to contribute to the DataDerm registry of the American Academy of Dermatology (AAD).[40–44]

In 2022, Bob was asked to assume the chair of the Department of Pathology. With the experience of running the Pathology Department as Interim chair for 22 months in 2017 and 2018, he took this job knowing that he would be spared from a dual chair role (dermatology and pathology) because Jeremy D. Jackson, MD, Vice Chair of the Department of Dermatology was ready to take on the role of dermatology chairperson. A person who just wanted to end his career in academics; who never thought he would have the opportunity to be a chair of a Department of Dermatology; was now ending his career as a Pathology chair. Both experiences proved to be tremendously gratifying and life-enriching.

## RECOMMENDATIONS
### Finding an Academic Mentor

Developing relationships with a primary mentor, and many other individuals who are willing to provide mentoring help throughout one's life, is essential to maximal achievement in any field. It is simply impossible to waste time and energy "reinventing the wheel" if one is going to make rapid progress toward goals. This story certainly demonstrates that effective guidance can help a "regular country boy" make special contributions to the field dermatology, his community, and most importantly to the success of students, residents, and colleagues. Then, mentoring others leads to something that may be unexpected. Mentees become colleagues and help their mentor in unexpected ways while they also begin to mentor the next generation.

### Set Small Measurable Goals

It would be tremendously frustrating to work toward end-of-career goals without setting small goals along the way. Thus, a private practitioner should think about getting an adjunct "volunteer" position at a medical school, perhaps then work to achieve a promotion to assistant professor, associate professor, and perhaps even become a clinical professor. Becoming a chairperson was an amazing combination of luck, serendipity, and timing that could never have been predicted.

### The Secret of Successful Individuals Is Helping Others

Adam Grant, Dean of the Wharton Business School at the University of Pennsylvania, wrote a tremendous book, *Give and Take*, that everyone should read.[45] It provides a number of vignettes and some scientific analysis concluding that the secret of successful individuals is "helping others." No one should engage in mentoring, teaching, succession planning, or other activities that help others *expecting* to be paid back! It is the just right thing to do. Then, you will find that the individuals around you contribute to your success in expected and quite unexpected ways.

### Learn and Practice Leadership Skills

Leadership is a learned skill. This talent comes from trial and error…. learning from one's mistakes. It also comes from study so that fewer errors need to be made.[28] **Table 1** lists several books that I have found helpful. The AAD also offers the AAD Leadership Institute, a leadership program with a special section for young academics (Academic Dermatology Leadership Program—ADLP) and an advanced program for individuals who have attained leadership positions in the academy. The AAD believes these programs help their organization but also believes these leadership skills lead to dermatologists being more effective community leaders… something that positions our field well in the House of Medicine.

They Said It Couldn't Be Done.

Early in Bob's career, a senior dermatologist in his community told him "You can be financially

**Table 1**
Recommended "self help" books for the private practitioner with a desire to end their career in academics

| Title | Author | Citation |
| --- | --- | --- |
| Give and Take: A Revolutionary Approach to Success[45] | Adam Grant | Grant A. *Give and Take a Revolutionary Approach to Success.* New York, NY: Viking; 2013 |
| How Doctors Think[46] | Jerome Groopman MD | Groopman JE. *How Doctors Think.* Boston: Houghton Mifflin; 2007. |
| Leaders Eat Last: Why Some Teams Pull Together and Others Don't[47] | Simon Sinek | Sinek S. *Leaders Eat Last: Why Some Teams Pull Together and Others Don't.* New York: Penguin Group; 2014. |
| Culture Trumps Everything: The Unexpected Truth About the Ways Environment Changes Biology Psychology and Behavior[48] | Gustavo R. Grodnitzky | Grodnitzky GR. *Culture Trumps Everything: The Unexpected Truth About the Ways Environment Changes Biology Psychology and Behavior.* Evergreen Colo: MountainFrog Publishing; 2014. |
| Start with Why: How Great Leaders Inspire Everyone to Take Action[49] | Simon Sinek | Sinek S. *Start with Why: How Great Leaders Inspire Everyone to Take Action.* New York: Portfolio/Penguin; 2011. |
| Think Again: The Power of Knowing What You Don't Know[50] | Adam Grant | Grant A. *Think Again: The Power of Knowing What You Don't Know.* New York New York: Viking an imprint of Penguin Random House LLC; 2021. |
| Originals: How Non-Conformists Move the World[51] | Adam Grant | Grant A. *Originals: How Non-Conformists Move the World.* New York New York: Penguin Books an imprint of Penguin Random House LLC; 2017. |
| Thinking, Fast and Slow[52] | Daniel Kahneman | Kahneman D. *Thinking Fast and Slow.* Toronto: Anchor Canada; 2013. |

successful or be an academic, but you can't be both." I used this as a motivating call to action. The enriched life we all strive to attain requires that one measure success in more than dollars earned.

## Keeping a Prospective Academic/Educator's Portfolio

Of all the things that can influence a career, this one may be the most important to an individual that may wish to end their career in academics. Promotion and tenure committees find it difficult to delineate quality in their assessments although they try hard. They are, however, very good at assessing quantity. Having a curriculum vitae (CV) or educator's portfolio listing every peer-reviewed publication, digital publication, membership, leadership

position, mentee, award, and much more is second nature to young academics but not to most private practicing dermatologists. It must be constructed in real time, prospectively. It is not difficult if one's administrative staff records the lectures you give, the medical students who rotate in your office, and so forth. It is also an amazing motivating tool as every listing is a way of recording "credit" for the work that has been accomplished.[11,12]

## Culture Trumps Everything

There is no book that had a greater impact on creating excellence than Gustavo Grodnitzky's book, "Culture Trumps Everything."[48] This book teaches leaders how to engender trust from team members and build a caring organization that is driven by more than a salary structure.

The investment in time and energy put into the development of a highly functioning culture pays rich dividends in the ability to hire and retain the best staff and improve patient satisfaction. It is the culture that makes Chick FilA function at a level much higher than McDonalds. Every individual in a leadership position should read this book.

### Find a Niche

It is impossible to do everything! Although there are some tasks you must complete because it is part of your job, it is important that you are passionate about the tasks you choose to enrich your life.[8] This provides the motivation to invest the hard work required to achieve goals. Selecting a special niche in dermatology or in a community activity outside of dermatology should be done carefully to harness this power. Mentors and experiences will help you to make important decisions about the niche's you wish to fill.

### Take Your Family with You on the Journey

The investment in time, money, and energy into one's work can be destructive to a family. "Family first" is a useful mantra. For most of us, without the support of family, it is much harder to be happy. For Dr Bob, when it was impossible to take the whole family, taking his wife or one of his children with him to a teaching venue, a hospital consultation, a national meeting, or a community event made these engagements much more enjoyable and provided special bonds and incredible memories. It also teaches children the importance of service and allows them to experience the warm feelings this engenders. It is worth the small amount of additional time required to plan for a sidekick accompanying you.

## FINAL WORDS

When asked to provide this article, my first reaction was that it would be impossible for anyone to provide advice based on one person's unique experiences. Perhaps because of my age, I took the opportunity to try. The final advice: do not settle. Do not settle for a life focused on 8 hours of work each day. Diversify your day to make it less like work! Do not settle for being a follower. Find passion in your life and allow it to guide you to lead. Do not settle for being like anyone else. Take a little advice from each teacher, each mentor, each family member, and become the individual who reached for special dreams, never worrying about falling short. We all fall short.

## CLINICS CARE POINTS

- Private practicing dermatologists can contribute to academic pursuits in their clinics.
- Transition to an academic career from private practice is possible with guidance from a mentor and planning

## CONFLICTS OF INTEREST

R.T. Brodell is a principal investigator for clinical trials (Novartis and Pfizer) the Corevitas psoriasis biologic registry, and owns stock in Veradermic, Inc. He serves on editorial boards of American Medical Student Research (faculty advisor); Practice Update Dermatology (Editor-in-Chief); Journal of the American Journal Academy of Dermatology (Associate Editor); Practical Dermatology; Journal of the Mississippi State Medical Society; SKIN: The Journal of Cutaneous Medicine and Archives of Dermatological Research.

## REFERENCES

1. Rajabi-Estarabadi A, Jones VA, Zheng C, et al. Dermatologist transitions: Academics into private practices and vice versa. Clin Dermatol 2020;38(5): 541–6.
2. Tso S. Potential barriers to pursuing a career in academic dermatology. Br J Dermatol 2016;175(1): 222–3.
3. Mezrich R, Nagy PG. The academic RVU: A system for measuring academic productivity. J Am Coll Radiol 2007;4(7):471–8.
4. Luong P, Bojansky AM, Kalra A. Academic physician compensation in the United States. Eur Heart J 2018;39(40):3633–4.
5. Bourne HR, Vermillion EB. Lost Dollars Threaten Research in Public Academic Health Centers. FASEB J 2017;31(3):863–85.
6. Meador KJ. Decline of clinical research in academic medical centers. Neurology 2015;85(13):1171–6.
7. Brodell RT. The role of the part-time physician-teacher in dermatology. Arch Dermatol 1996;132(7): 758.
8. Developing your professional niche as an academic clinician-educator. ASCO Connection. https://connection.asco.org/blogs/developing-your-professional-niche-academic-clinician-educator. Published October 1, 2020. Accessed August 17, 2022.
9. Brodell RT. Do more than discuss that unusual case. PGM (Postgrad Med) 2000;108(2):19–23.

10. Brodell RT. Learning and teaching in dermatology. A practitioner's guide. Arch Dermatol 1996;132(8): 946–52.

11. Saltman DC, Tavabie A, Kidd MR. The use of reflective and reasoned portfolios by doctors. J Eval Clin Pract 2010;18(1):182–5.

12. Brodell RT, Alam M, Bickers DR. The dermatologist's academic portfolio. Am J Clin Dermatol 2003;4(11):733–6.

13. Brodell RT, Helms SE. Remaining a Great Physician in Tough Times: Learning from Business Principles. Journal of the Mississippi Medical Society 2014 55;(7):239–40.

14. Rush JL, Helms SE, Mostow EN. The CARE approach to reducing diagnostic errors. Int J Dermatol 2017;56(6):669–73.

15. The duties of a doctor registered with the General Medical Council https://www.gmc-uk.org/ethical-guidance/ethical-guidance-for-doctors/good-medical-practice/duties-of-a-doctor. Accessed August 22, 2022.

16. Brodell RT. Letter to the Editor: The fundamental duties of the physician. Academic Medicine Journal 2000;75(12):1149–50.

17. Brodell RT. The two fundamental duties of the physician? Acad Med 2000;75(12):1149–50.

18. Helms AE, Helms SE, Brodell RT. Hospital consultations: Time to address an unmet need? J Am Acad Dermatol 2009;60(2):308–11.

19. Dunbar M, Helms SE, Brodell RT. Reducing cognitive errors in dermatology: Can anything be done? J Am Acad Dermatol 2013;69(5):810–3.

20. Helms SE, Brodell RT. Let's acknowledge our mistakes and learn from them. Br J Dermatol 2018; 179(6):1237–9.

21. Poulos GA, Brodell RT, Mostow EN. Improving quality and patient satisfaction in Dermatology Office Practice. Arch Dermatol 2008;144(2). https://doi.org/10.1001/archdermatol.2007.58.

22. Julia Burke AE. The symbiotic mentor/mentee relationship. DVM 360. https://www.dvm360.com/view/the-symbiotic-mentor-mentee-relationship, 2022. Accessed August 21, 2022.

23. Toklu HZ, Fuller JC. Mentor-mentee relationship: A win-win contract in Graduate Medical Education. Cureus 2017. https://doi.org/10.7759/cureus.1908.

24. Bauça JM. Reflections on the Mentor-Mentee Relationship: A Symbiosis. EJIFCC 2018;29(3):230–3.

25. Brodell R. Academic medicine in private practice. American Medical Student Research Journal 2014; 1(S1):1–6.

26. Fleming I, Eyre H, Pogue J, Bush GHW. Chapter 7: Victory Laps, . The American Cancer Society: A History of Saving Lives. The American Cancer Society; 2009. p. 133–7.

27. Gordon PA, Gordon BA. The role of volunteer organizations in leadership skill development. J Manag Dev 2017;36(5):712–23.

28. Brodell MDRT, Brodell DW. Storytelling in dermatology. SKIN The Journal of Cutaneous Medicine 2019;3(5):366–7.

29. Kindley KJ, Jackson JD, Sisson WT. Improving dermatology clinical efficiency in academic medical centers. Int J Health Sci 2015;9(3):347–50.

30. Straka BT, Wiser TH, Feldman SR, et al. The clinical triage assistant: A new member of the Dermatology Health Care Team. J Am Acad Dermatol 2010;63(6): 1103–5.

31. Streifel A, Wessman LL, Farah RS, et al. Rural residency curricula: Potential Target for improved access to care? Cutis 2021;107(1). https://doi.org/10.12788/cutis.0149.

32. Uhlenhake E, Brodell R, Mostow E. The Dermatology Work Force: A focus on urban versus Rural Wait Times. J Am Acad Dermatol 2009;61(1):17–22.

33. Fabbro SK, Mostow EN, Helms SE, et al. The pharmacist role in Dermatologic Care. Currents in Pharmacy Teaching and Learning 2014;6(1):92–105.

34. Lewiecki EM, Rochelle R. Project ECHO: Telehealth to Expand Capacity to Deliver Best Practice Medical Care. Rheum Dis Clin North Am 2019;45(2):303–14.

35. Bhate C, Ho CH, Brodell RT. Time to revisit the Health Insurance Portability and Accountability Act (HIPAA)? Accelerated telehealth adoption during the COVID-19 pandemic. J Am Acad Dermatol 2020 Oct;83(4):e313–4.

36. Pearlman RL, Brodell RT, Byrd AC. Enhancing access to rural Dermatological Care. JAMA Dermatology 2022;158(7):725.

37. Gronbeck C, Kodumudi V, Brodell RT, et al. Dermatology Workforce in the United States - Part 1: Overview, Transformations, and Implications. J Am Acad Dermatol 2022. S0190-9622(22)02240-X.

38. Kodumudi V, Gronbeck C, Brodell RT, et al. Dermatology Workforce in the United States: Part II - Patient Outcomes, Challenges, and Potential Solutions. J Am Acad Dermatol 2022. https://doi.org/10.1016/j.jaad.2022.06.1192. S0190-9622(22)02241-1.

39. Brodell RT, Byrd AC, Firkins-Smith C, et al, editors. Dermatology in rural settings: organizational, clinical, and Socioeconomic Perspectives. Sustainable development goals Series. Cham, Switzerland: Springer Nature; 2021.

40. Saul K, Casamiquela K, McCowan N, et al. The Clinical Learning Environment Review as a model for impactful self-directed quality control initiatives in Clinical Practice. Cutis 2016;97(2):96–100.

41. Morrissette S, Etkin CD, Brodell RT, et al. The Use of Clinical Data Registries to Improve Care and Meet Ongoing Professional Practice Evaluation Requirements. Jt Comm J Qual Patient Saf 2022. https://doi.org/10.1016/j.jcjq.2022.06.003. S1553-7250(22)00122-2.

42. Morrissette S, Pearlman RL, Kovar M, et al. Attitudes and perceived barriers toward store-and-forward

teledermatology among primary care providers of the rural Mississippi. Arch Dermatol Res 2021. https://doi.org/10.1007/s00403-021-02208-z.

43. Spell CA, Pearlman RL, Brodell RT, et al. Teledermatology Before and After CPVID-19: The Impact of Regulation. J Miss State Med Assoc (Special Edition: COVID-19 in Mississippi: Lessons Learned at UMMC). 2020, 61(11): 418-421.

44. Pearlman RL, Le PB, Brodell RT, et al. Evaluation of patient attitudes towards the technical experience of synchronous teledermatology in the era of COVID-19. Arch Dermatol Res 2021;13(9):769–72.

45. Grant A. Give and take a Revolutionary approach to success. New York, NY: Viking; 2013.

46. Groopman JE. How Doctors think. Boston: Houghton Mifflin; 2007.

47. Sinek S. Leaders Eat Last : Why some teams Pull Together and others Don't. New York: Penguin Group; 2014.

48. Grodnitzky GR. Culture Trumps everything : the unexpected Truth about the ways Environment changes Biology Psychology and Behavior. Evergreen Colo: MountainFrog Publishing; 2014.

49. Sinek S. Start with Why : how great leaders Inspire everyone to take action. New York: Portfolio/Penguin; 2011.

50. Grant A. Think Again: the Power of knowing what you Don't know. New York New York: Viking an imprint of Penguin Random House LLC; 2021.

51. Grant A. Originals : how Non-Conformists move the World. New York New York: Penguin Books an imprint of Penguin Random House LLC; 2017.

52. Kahneman D. Thinking Fast and Slow. Toronto: Anchor Canada; 2013.

# Political Activism and the Dermatologist

Martha Laurin Council, MD, MBA[a], George J. Hruza, MD, MBA[b,c],*

## KEYWORDS

• Advocacy • Activism • Legislation • Health policy • Public service

## KEY POINTS

- The dermatologist can help shape policy, which affects the practice of medicine.
- Maintaining a relationship with your state and federal legislators is paramount toward this end.
- Involvement in organized medicine can facilitate the physician-legislator relationship.

## INTRODUCTION

Dermatology, being an extremely competitive specialty to get into residency, selects for the brightest physicians. Traditionally, professionalism is thought of as taking excellent care of our patients leaving advocacy for health care policy to others. The health care industry is the most regulated industry. Taking excellent care of our patients is very important, but we need to look beyond our office/clinic to fully live up to our professional calling. We have a duty to advocate for our patients' safety, access to quality care, and for the continued ability to care for our patients. The practice of dermatology is governed by legislation and regulations at the local, state, and federal levels, including via state medical licensing boards, Health and Human Services regulations, private insurer policies, and by legislation. Although advocacy makes up very little of our training in medical school and residency, it is a critical component of safeguarding our ability to practice medicine and to protect our patients. If we are not at the table, we will be on the menu (Fig. 1).

Legislators, namely state and federal senators and representatives, tend to have very little knowledge of the practice of medicine and, often unintended, the consequences of laws that they pass. Maintaining an open dialogue with these legislators is important so that they can put into effect policy that will protect patients and our specialty. For dermatologists new to advocacy, starting this process may seem daunting. With the help of local and state medical societies as well as national specialty organizations, the process of advocating for our patients and specialty can be facilitated (Table 1).

## DISCUSSION

As a practicing dermatologist, one of the most important facets of our job is to protect the safety of our patients. Whether promoting a public health initiative such as the use of sunscreen and sun-protective clothing in schools, supporting truth in advertising, or promoting proper supervision of physician extenders, the dermatologist is in the unique position of being on the front lines of the physician–patient relationship. The dermatologist has unique insight into issues and a great understanding of what is at hand and, as such, can be a tremendous resource for policy makers. It is therefore critical that we continuously advocate for our patients (Fig. 2).

Disclosure: M.L. Council has served as a consultant for Abbvie, Castle Biosciences, and Regeneron. G.J. Hruza has been a candidate for Missouri State Senate and chair of the American Academy of Dermatology Association's SkinPAC[1] Board of Advisors.

[a] Washington University in St. Louis, 969 North Mason Road, Suite 200, St Louis, MO 63141, USA; [b] Laser & Dermatologic Surgery Center, 1001 Chesterfield Parkway East, Suite 101, Chesterfield, MO 63017, USA; [c] St. Louis University
* Corresponding author. Laser & Dermatologic Surgery Center, and St. Louis University, 1001 Chesterfield Parkway East, Suite 101, Chesterfield, MO 63017.
E-mail address: ghruza@gmail.com

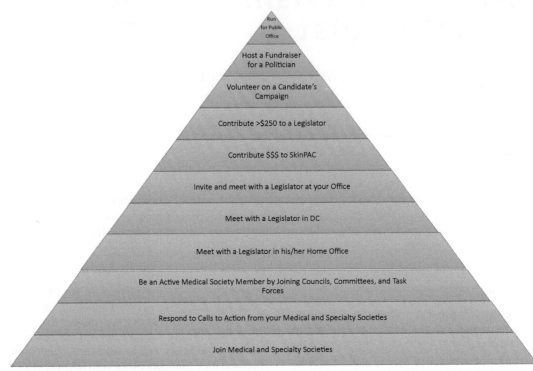

**Fig. 1.** Pyramid of advocacy involvement.

**Table 1**
**Dos and Don'ts of advocacy**

| Do | Don't |
|---|---|
| Familiarize yourself with issues currently affecting the practice of medicine. | Worry that you aren't an expert on policy or the legislative branch. You are an expert in your specialty and a patient-advocate. |
| Bring impactful stories to show how patients are affected by policy or lack thereof. | Focus solely on the physician, but rather on how policy affects our ability to care for our patients. |
| Dress professionally. If you are advocating as part of a group, you may wear your white coat as a symbol of your profession. | Be overly casual; you are representing your specialty. |
| Be organized and have three to four concrete "asks." | Be disorganized or vague in your requests. |
| Try to meet with your representatives at least annually to build a relationship over time. | Decline to meet with staffers or to meet virtually if this is all that is offered. Staff members inform the legislators and you can have a meaningful relationship with them, too. |
| Meet with legislators from any political party. Thank those who have given you support in the past and persuade those who haven't. | Be tied to a particular political party. You are representing your specialty, and you need the support of legislators from all parties. |
| Leave your succinct asks in writing after the meeting so your legislator has something to refer to. | Forget to thank your legislator for his/her time. |

The pyramid (Fig. 1) contains the following levels from bottom to top:
- Join Medical and Specialty Societies
- Respond to Calls to Action from your Medical and Specialty Societies
- Be an Active Medical Society Member by Joining Councils, Committees, and Task Forces
- Meet with a Legislator in his/her Home Office
- Meet with a Legislator in DC
- Invite and meet with a Legislator at your Office
- Contribute $$$ to SkinPAC
- Contribute >$250 to a Legislator
- Volunteer on a Candidate's Campaign
- Host a Fundraiser for a Politician
- Run for Public Office

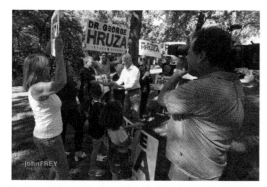

**Fig. 2.** George Hruza, MD MBA, runs for Missouri State Senate. (*Courtesy of* Frey J, St. Louis, MO.)

In addition, we dermatologists must advocate for our specialty to preserve the practice of medicine for our colleagues in generations to come. Threats to this practice come in many forms: burdensome regulatory tasks that do not improve patient outcomes, cuts to Medicare and Medicaid spending that could limit patient access and/or our ability to keep our doors open for our patients, and unfunded administrative burdens such as prior authorization and step therapy processes that delay or inhibit our ability to care for our patients. It is so important for dermatologists to communicate to policy makers exactly what these threats are so that they can be mitigated.

Naturally, dermatologists must have a means of opening the lines of communication with policy makers to assure that our voice is heard. Maintaining regular correspondence with state and federal legislators is an important part of assuring that the dermatologists' voice is heard. There are several ways in which this dialogue can occur, but email, phone, and in person are the three most common means.

Legislators want to hear from those they serve. Constituents are voters, and voters determine whether or not a legislator will be reelected for another term. Should a dermatologist want the support of a policy maker on a particular bill, for example, he or she could simply draft a brief email to said policy maker outlining the request. Such messages carry additional weight when they are supported by patient anecdotes or meaningful stories which can further support the request. On receiving an email, the legislator or staff member will typically issue a response and makes a notation of issues which garner particular interest. Our professional organizations will send out alerts to take action on pressing issues that are being debated in the legislature, such as Medicare reimbursement cuts, with a pre-templated email that is linked to the specific dermatologist's member of Congress and Senators. The more such emails legislators receive

on the issue, the better chance of seeing action. These email templates have room for a personal story about how the legislation will affect one's practice and patients. It is important to take advantage of the opportunity to personalize these emails. Even though these email alerts are very easy to respond to and take action, consistently, only about 15% of dermatologists respond.

The next step up the ladder of influence is a personal phone call to your legislator. Legislators are amenable to phone conversations with constituents on important issues. Should a topic require further dialogue, a dermatologist can request a phone or electronic meeting with the policy maker or a staff member. It is important to keep asking clear and succinct and to be prepared for questions which may arise during the conversation.

A personal meeting with a legislator and/or their staff on issues that are important tends to have more impact than calls or emails. Legislators appreciate that you consider the issue important enough to close your office to meet with them. Requests to meet can often be scheduled online. The meetings can occur in your office, in the legislator's home office ("district office"), or in their state/federal legislative office. By meeting with legislators regularly, on an annual or semiannual basis, one can create meaningful long-term relationships. It is important to try to remain nonpartisan during such meetings and to approach the conversation from the point of view of what would be best for the patient and specialty, regardless of the legislator's political party affiliation. The American Academy of Dermatology Association (AADA)[2] has an annual fly-in to Washington, DC where dermatologists learn about advocacy, and how to be an effective advocate for dermatology issues and then the attendees swarm onto "the Hill" in small groups to advocate with legislators from their home state (**Fig. 3**). These meetings last about 20 to 30 minutes each and are usually with the legislator or their health care legislative assistant. Other dermatology organizations also set up these fly-ins. Since the pandemic, these are sometimes virtual. Many state medical societies have annual legislative "white coat" days where physicians across the state come to the state capital to advocate with their legislators (**Fig. 4**). Both the Washington, DC fly-ins and state white coat days can deliver a powerful message about how important we find various health care issues. They are only effective if we can muster a large number of physicians to participate.

Politics boils down to voters and dollars. Those that can provide the most voters and/or most dollars tend to get the ear of the legislator. Legislators appreciate having financial support. Running a

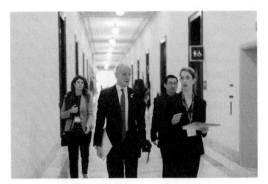

**Fig. 3.** American Academy of Dermatology Association Legislative Conference.

political campaign is a very costly process, and constituents who contribute financially toward the election or reelection of a legislator will have a louder voice. When considering a contribution to a legislator, one should be strategic to maximize the impact of the contribution. Contributions are all about relationship-building (**Fig. 5**). The best time to contribute to a candidate is early in the campaign or, in a hotly contested race, toward the end of the campaign. The contribution should be in person at a fundraising event whenever possible so that you have the possibility to get to know the legislator in person and vice versa. For federal office, contributions of $250 or more are reported to the Federal Election Commission with differing thresholds for state legislators. Giving at or above the threshold means that when you meet with the legislator at a later date, they are likelier to be aware of your financial support. Of course, one also needs to be aware of the various limits on contributions and that political contributions are not deductible as either a charitable contribution or as a business expenses. In most jurisdictions, money given directly to candidates has to be made with personal funds. The next step up the ladder of impact is to hold a fundraiser for your legislator. Getting all your friends together to support your legislator takes a lot of legwork, but the legislator will be very grateful (well, at least until

the next election, when they will be asking what have you done for them lately).

To leverage dermatology's advocacy impact, the AADA sets up a political action committee more than two decades ago: SkinPAC. SkinPAC accepts contributions form AADA members that are disbursed to federal candidates for the House and Senate to support their campaigns. SkinPAC uses a scorecard based on how the candidate stands on AADA priorities. The higher the score, the more money the candidate's campaign becomes eligible for. Points are also assigned based on the legislator's ability to influence legislation important for our specialty such as being in leadership or on a key committee (eg, Energy and Commerce in the House). SkinPAC is a nonpartisan PAC distributing funds in a bipartisan manner with distributions to democrats and republicans divided close to 50/50. The generosity of about 15% of AADA members has raised a record amount, since its founding, during the 2021 to 2022 election cycle. SkinPAC is now the fourth largest medical specialty Political Action

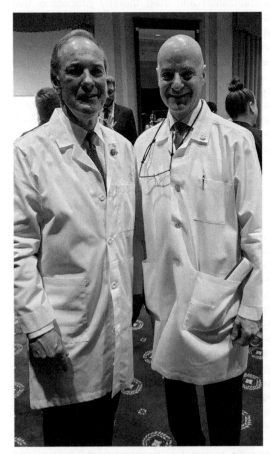

**Fig. 5.** Representative Dr John Joyce and Dr George Hruza at a skin cancer screening event on Capitol Hill.

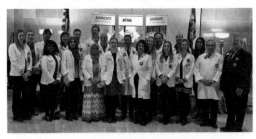

**Fig. 4.** Missouri State Medical Association white coat day.

Committee (PAC). SkinPAC is a key tool for the AADA Washington office, the AADA Congressional Policy Committee, and the sister societies (American Society of Dermatologic Surgery Association [ASDSA],[3] American College of Mohs Surgery [ACMS], and American Society of Mohs Surgery) to work with legislators on issues of importance to our patients and practices. Should you live in a district or state where your legislator(s) is of the opposite party and you prefer to not contribute to them directly, SkinPAC is a great way to contribute to legislators of both main parties that support dermatology issues without getting caught up in the partisan issues that are so prevalent today.

The American Medical Association (AMA)[4] has a PAC as do many state medical societies and even some state dermatology societies. Support of the PAC in your state is important as many of the issues affecting our day-to-day practice are decided at the state level. The good thing is that, at the state level, a little money goes a long way. A $100 contribution to a state legislator will go a lot further than a $1000 contribution to a federal legislator.

The bridge between the practicing dermatologist and the policy maker can often be facilitated by local and state medical societies and by our national specialty organizations. Local and state medical societies can help one to remain abreast of policies being introduced at the local and state levels. These organizations are made up of physicians from many specialties and often organize advocacy days at the state capital and/or meetings with state senators and representatives. Many specialty societies and the AMA offer model bills that one can suggest to state legislators on issues that affect our patients and practices. Specialty societies often encourage in person visits when federal legislators are back in their districts during legislative recess. These societies will provide talking points and specific asks and will facilitate scheduling of visits, essentially streamlining the process for busy clinicians. In addition to being a member of your specialty organizations and state and local societies, you can increase your input and advocacy efforts by joining committees dealing with advocacy and ultimately run for office in these organizations (**Box 1**). AADA, ASDSA, and ACMS all have leadership training programs that can be helpful in getting your foot in the door. Being actively involved in organized medicine and ultimately ascend to leadership, you can leverage your personal advocacy efforts to new heights. To be able to continue to offer the excellent care for our patients, we all have to become more involved in advocacy to whatever level we are able.

---

**Box 1**
**Advocacy Priorities of the American Academy of Dermatology, 2023.**

- Medicare Payment Reform that establishes a positive annual inflation adjustment, replaces or eliminates the budget neutrality requirements of the physician fee schedule, and reforms the Quality Payment Program to increase physician input and improve patient care without overly burdensome documentation and compliance activity.

- Develop patient-centered models of care that assure accurate and sustainable reimbursement, strengthen relationships with other specialties within the house of medicine to provide coordinated patient care, and clarify the roles of board-certified dermatologists and non-physician clinicians in the care team.

- Promote access to care by fellows of the American Academy of Dermatology, particularly in underserved areas.

*Adapted from* American Academy of Dermatology Association. ACADEMY ADVOCACY PRIORITIES. Available at: https://www.aad.org/member/advocacy/priorities/advocacy-priorities. Accessed Jan 24 2023.

---

If you have done all of the foregoing and still want to have more impact in the legislative and regulatory process, you can try to get appointed to your state medical board (usually a political process) or run for public office. Many state legislatures are part-time (eg, Texas legislature meets only every other year), so one can continue to practice dermatology at least part-time when in state elective office. A state medical board position should have minimal impact on day-to-day dermatology practice. Federal legislative office is more along the line of a new career as one cannot have an outside remunerated job. If you are interested in public service, the AMA has a weekend candidate workshop and a weeklong campaign school. The ASDSA also has a program for members aspiring to serve on medical boards or in public office. If you do decide to run for public office, be prepared for an inspiring, energizing, expensive, all-encompassing, exhausting, and exhilarating experience.

## SUMMARY

In conclusion, it is important that the dermatologist serves as a liaison between the patient and government on issues that affect patient safety and the physician's ability to practice medicine. Building and maintaining a relationship with legislators at all levels of government are critical toward maintaining the physician's voice, and local and state medical societies as well as national specialty organizations can simplify this process.

## CLINICS CARE POINTS

- The dermatologist has a professional responsibility of advocating for our specialty and patients.
- One can interface with state and federal legislators on issues impacting our specialty via email, phone, or in-person meetings.
- Local and state medical societies, national specialty societies, and the American Medical Association are resources for all physicians aspiring to be more involved in organized medicine.

## REFERENCES

1. AMERICAN ACADEMY OF DERMATOLOGY ASSOCIATION POLITICAL ACTION COMMITTEE. Available at: https://www.skinpac.org. Accessed January 24 2023.

2. American Academy of Dermatology Association. ADVOCACY. Available at: https://www.aad.org/member/advocacy. Accessed January 24 2023.

3. American Society for Dermatologic Surgery Association. DEDICATED TO ADVOCACY ON BEHALF OF DERMATOLOGIC SURGEONS AND THEIR PATIENTS. Available at: https://www.asds.net/asdsa-advocacy. Accessed January 24 2023.

4. American Medical Association. Available at: https://www.ama-assn.org. Accessed January 24 2023.

# How to Be a Successful Businesswoman in Dermatology

Cyndi Yag-Howard, MD, FAAD

## KEYWORDS

- Business • Businesswoman • Success • Successful • Practice

## KEY POINTS

- Success is a personal construct.
- The intent of this article is to help the reader formulate their own vision of success and to provide advice to get the reader on their own road to success.
- The content of the article is based on interviews with many successful businesswomen in dermatology, as well as the personal experience of the author.

## INTRODUCTION

Success is a personal construct. The intent of this article is to help you formulate your vision of success and offer advice to get you on your own road to success.[1] It is based on personal experience as well as interviews with many successful businesswomen in dermatology whom I have had the good fortune of befriending over the years. It is hoped that, some or most of these ideas, thoughts, and suggestions resonate with you and can help you on your journey.

## DISCUSSION
### What Is Success?

#### Define success
The first step to becoming a successful businesswoman or businessperson in dermatology, or in any field for that matter, is to define what success means to you.[2] For some, success equals wealth or fame. For others, it means autonomy, knowledge, favorable patient outcomes, balance, happiness in the workplace, good stewardship, or any number of other concepts.

For me, I was driven by a desire for autonomy and balance that would allow me the flexibility to spend meaningful time with my family and the freedom to stay engaged in organized medicine. It was important to me to be able to grow and build the brand of my solo private dermatology practice while also making a difference for our specialty and our patients. I was also driven by a desire for excellence. I knew that if I were to start a practice, it had to offer exceptional care in a uniquely friendly and caring environment that would exceed patient expectations—the type of atmosphere that I would most enjoy as a patient. In these areas, I feel I have succeeded. Yet, my vision of success changes as I move through life. As I begin to feel comfortable and balanced on one stepping stone, I set my sights on the next direction and stepping stone along the way. Success to me is fluid, dynamic, and accompanied by a sense of satisfaction, gratitude, and fulfillment.

#### Realize success has different meanings to different people
In the words of Kavita Mariwalla, MD, owner of Mariwalla Dermatology in New York and Vice President of the American Society for Dermatologic Surgeons (ASDS), "In dermatology, success has meant being able to grow and build something that results in better patient care. Everything I have added to my practice in terms of services or technology has always had that in mind. It's not so much 'will it make me money', but rather 'will this improve patient care or allow us to be able to offer something we don't already have?' My father

University of South Florida Morsani College of Medicine, Yag-Howard Cosmetic Dermatology, 1000 Goodlette Road, Suite 100, Naples, FL 34102, USA
E-mail address: drcyndi@yhderm.com

Dermatol Clin 41 (2023) 659–666
https://doi.org/10.1016/j.det.2023.07.002
0733-8635/23/© 2023 Elsevier Inc. All rights reserved.

always says, 'Don't chase money, let money chase you'. So keeping patients in the forefront of what decisions I make has been the marker of success for me" (e-mail communication, February 2023).

To other successful businesswomen in dermatology, success has to do with patient outcomes and the work environment. According to Melissa Piliang, MD, Associate Professor of Dermatology, Vice Chair of Education, and Co-Director of Dermatopathology Sections at Cleveland Clinic, Cleveland, Ohio, "My personal definition of success is making things better–patients, processes, mentees. Because, for me, that is what it is all about–caring for patients, helping people. When someone recognizes that something I did helped them, the feeling I get is indescribable–it feels like success" (e-mail communication, February 2023).

To others, success has to do with leadership. For Cheryl Burgess, MD, founder of the Center for Dermatology and Dermatologic Surgery in Washington, DC, and former member of the AAD Board of Directors, "You know when you're successful (in dermatology and in life) when you become a leader amongst those in your environment or surroundings; everything appears effortless and there is a sense of calmness that fulfils your well-being. A leader looks for opportunities to give of themselves freely to others rather than holding back; build rather than tear down; serve rather than be served and be willing to learn and remain teachable to pass it forward" (e-mail communication, January 2023).

To Doris Day, MD, author, medical consultant, and owner of Day Dermatology and Aesthetics in New York, success is dynamic. "I think of success as an ongoing process, not an end. It's something I see looking back and something I strive for daily as I go forward, but it's not something I have in the moment. It sums up as loving what I do and feeling fulfilled by the life I am living. I want to look back and live a life that I would live the same way over and over again; that would be a great success. It's something I try to live by every day" (e-mail communication, January 2023). Like Dr Day, Deirdre Hooper, MD, cofounder of Audubon Dermatology in New Orleans and treasurer of ASDS, sees success broadly. "I feel most successful when I am enjoying the people around me–my family, my colleagues, and my work team. Of course, I love setting and achieving a goal, but I have learned to set goals that feed a balanced family life and satisfy my intellectual curiosity. The rest just seems to follow" (e-mail communication, February 2023). And to internationally renowned oculoplastic surgeon and honorary

lifetime member of the American Academy of Dermatology (AAD), Jean Carruthers, MD, whose entrepreneurial spirit led to the first use of botulinum toxin as a neuromodulator, success is simple. "Success to me means I am liked and respected by my peers and my patients and students!" (text message communication, February 2023).

Other successful businesswomen in dermatology believe that success is achieved when one finds balance. According to Mona Gohara, MD, medical consultant and President of the Women's Dermatologic Society, "To me, success is finding fulfillment and balance in your professional and personal life. There is nothing greater than enjoying life in and out of the office" (e-mail communication, January 2023). Similarly, Sue Ellen Cox, MD, founder and medical director of Aesthetic Solutions in North Carolina and Immediate Past President of ASDS, says, "An important aspect of success for many is a balanced life–physical, mental and spiritual. It is also important to contribute to your specialty and pay forward all the success and privileges that you have been given" (e-mail communication, January 2023).

## How to Become Successful

### Decide what type of practice you really want

Today, your practice model options are relatively limitless.[3] You can be a subspecialist, an academician or private practitioner, an owner or an employee, or any combination of the aforementioned. If you aren't sure, it's ok. You can always change your track. However, the sooner you head down your chosen path, the sooner and more fully you will be able to develop and grow your career.

Perhaps the 2 most important decisions to make early on are whether you want to pursue an academic, nonacademic, or combination of academic and private practice career and whether you want to be a business owner or an employee.[4,5] The time commitments associated with any of these paths can be quite variable, as is the level of responsibility one assumes.

Personally, I chose the path of being the owner of a solo private practice with an academic affiliation. This choice enabled me to teach residents and remain connected with my academic institution while allowing me the opportunity to build my own practice model and provide the type of personalized care that is very important to me. Being a practice owner means that I am essentially responsible not only for the care of my patients but also for the livelihood and well-being of my entire staff; 24/7/365, everything that occurs within the walls of my practice is my responsibility. I am willing to accept that responsibility because autonomy is very important to me, and owning a solo practice aligns with that priority. Essentially, if you align your business with your life, you can achieve happiness, which I believe to be a major contributor to success.

### Align your business with your life

Determine your priorities and make sure that your practice aligns with those priorities. For some people, financial remuneration is a priority and a major contributing factor in why they choose their career path. Understand that compensation varies greatly depending on the career path you choose in dermatology. Niche specialization and/or a concierge type of practice may yield higher compensation than an academic, rural, or part-time practice. Interestingly, not one successful businesswoman in dermatology whom I interviewed mentioned money or identified it with success.

For many dermatologists, location is a priority. Do you want to live near your extended family, near a major academic center, or in a remote underserved area? Do you want to travel and undertake a locum tenens position? Or do you want to live wherever you find your dream job? Also consider your commute. If you have or plan to have a family, obviously a longer commute equates to less time with family. And if time is your priority, owning a solo practice or running an academic program will likely yield significantly less free time than job-sharing or working part-time in an established clinic.

### Choose your work and home locations wisely

When making sure that the life you create is the life you want, location becomes very important. If snow skiing is one of your greatest sources of exercise and enjoyment, you probably won't want to live in a warm climate. If you thrive off fast-paced hustle and bustle, you probably won't want to work in a rural town far from a city. Since you will likely spend much of your time working, having the ability to escape to your happy place during those brief interludes of time will be important.

The location of your work in relation to your home is also extremely important. Long commutes can be stressful and hard on you, your significant other, and your family. The more time you spend traveling means the less time you get to spend with the ones you love—the ones who support you and need you.

If you have children, the distance from your work to your school system matters. Working close to your children's school system will allow you the chance to attend school activities, sporting events, performances, and so on and be readily available if your children need you. My husband, Corey Howard, MD, and I chose to live near our workplace so that we could maximize family time and be readily available to head back to the office in the event of a patient emergency. In fact, availability and flexibility were important factors that led us to become solo private practice owners.

### Whatever practice type you choose, make a plan

Whether you decide to open your own practice by yourself or with others, join an established practice, or enter academic medicine, there are innumerable online resources that can assist you in the process.[6,7] In addition, the American Academy of Dermatology (AAD) offers many resources to help you in your career path. For instance, the AAD Practice Resource Center offers valuable online and hard copy tools to help you regardless of what type of practice you enter.[8] They also have staff dedicated to answering your practice management questions whether you are just starting your practice or are well-established in your career.

If you start a dermatology practice, it will be a much different experience if you start it on your own versus starting it with others. If you start your own independent practice, you have the luxury of making all your decisions but also the responsibility of assuming all the risks.[9] Before going into business with others, make sure your vision, goals, and expectations align. It is helpful if your strengths and weaknesses complement each other in a way that will help ensure practice viability.

As Deanne Mraz Robinson, MD, President and Co-founder of Modern Dermatology of Connecticut and Chief Medical Officer of Ideal Image, says, "Business success means financial, intellectual and operational freedom. I achieved this by opening my own practice with my partner. We created a work culture that not only emphasized patient care, but also stressed the well-being of the provider to focus on work-life balance." Although their visions aligned, before establishing their partnership, Dr Mraz Robinson and her business partner engaged in the all-important step of writing and signing a contract. "We wrote our contract as if we were dissolving the practice before we even opened the doors. We prepared for the worst so we could be ready for whatever happened" (text message communication, February 2023).

Starting a practice requires making a business plan.[4] It will help you critically analyze what your goals are, what resources you need to achieve those initial goals, what it will cost you, what steps you must take, and what nuances you might encounter as you develop your business. You will need to share your business plan with your bank or lending partner if you are getting funding.[6] I recommend getting lending quotes from several banks before deciding on one. Banks might compete for better loan rates that may be fixed versus adjustable, long-term, or short-term. If possible, make sure that there is minimal or no penalty for early pay-off, which you may want to do, if financially feasible, to avoid paying additional interest.

### Surround yourself with the right people

Regardless of what practice type you choose, it is important to find the professionals who will help you manage important aspects of your life.[9] They include your lawyer, accountant, banker, advisor, and insurer. When seeking out these professionals, do not hesitate to ask them if they can recommend experts in the other fields. The better they know you, your practice or professional circumstances, and your financial situation, the more helpful (and possibly less expensive) they will be. Meeting with them on an annual or semiannual basis will ensure accuracy of your accounts and finances and ensure that you are prepared for the future. Having their contact information at your fingertips will help alleviate stress when time is of the essence. There might even be benefit in building connections between them. For instance, when seeking advice about borrowing money for the purchase or lease of a laser or other expensive device, you might want your financial lender to connect with your accountant or financial advisor so that their expertise contributes favorably to your decision-making.

As the business owner of my own dermatology practice, I realized early on that, in addition to the aforementioned professionals, I needed to hire a good office administrator to help me manage my business. I knew that I could not manage my office administration, financials, human resources, patient services, communications, marketing, and everything else it takes to run an office without the help of someone who knew how to do these tasks better than I did. Unfortunately, my first administrator did not work out well. Nor did my second. Nor third. Finding the right practice administrator is perhaps the most difficult part of operating a business. Physicians are notorious for being "bad at business," so we are ripe targets for being taken advantage of financially. My practice was no exception.

I found that applicants seeking an office administrator position frequently overstate their qualifications and are unable to meet the needs of the job. Thankfully, my husband, who is also a physician, but who manages to grasp business concepts better than most, was able to pull my business through the tough times when I was "between" office administrators. Although difficult to do, making the time, energy, and financial investment to obtain the right administrator is critical. Your administrator can make or break your practice. I recommend hiring an administrator who has an MBA or equivalent experience, a keen business acumen, and a vision that is in keeping with your goals. Meet with your administrator at least weekly to review staffing issues and day-to-day operations, at least monthly to review financials (balance sheet, profit and loss statements, income and spending trends, etc.), and at least biannually to review budget, marketing needs, and long-term goals.

### Delegate appropriately

Many, if not most, physicians are strong-minded and driven self-starters who are not used to relying on others. To be successful in the business of dermatology means you must rely on others by delegating responsibilities wisely and regularly—both at work and at home. You might be the type to say that if you want the job done right, you have to do it yourself. However, as your responsibilities and time demands increase, especially if you have a family at home, you will find that you simply cannot do everything yourself. You must give up the reigns of total control and delegate.

Most importantly, delegate the jobs you don't like doing and the jobs you don't need to do to someone else. Hiring people to help with cleaning and cooking, for instance, can give you the gift of time to spend with your family or to use for work, exercise, or mental health. The money you spend will pay for itself in your increased happiness and productivity.

At work, let people you trust and who are capable of doing things for you do them. For instance, if you are used to doing your own anesthesia for a biopsy, but your nurse is proficient at numbing, let them anesthetize the patient. If your aesthetic patient wants to know about postprocedure care and your staff is well-versed in it, let them answer the questions. Essentially, find people you trust to do the things you don't like to do or don't have to do, and you will have more time for doing the things that matter most to you.

### Accept support

Undoubtedly, successful businesswomen share one thing in common—the support of others who helped them reach their goals. Support can come in many different forms—offering advice, boosting confidence, assisting financially, providing guidance, sharing knowledge or contacts, and so on. In whatever form it comes, appreciate the support you receive and accept the support you might need.

As Adelaide Hebert, MD, Past President of both Women's Dermatological Society and the Society of Pediatric Dermatology, as well as Chief of Pediatric Dermatology at McGovern School of Medicine and Children's Memorial Hermann Hospital in Houston, says, "I feel that I became a successful businesswoman in Dermatology because my father (an obstetrician gynecologist) treated all of his seven children equally and genuinely believed that his girls would be as well-educated and prepared for life as his boys." She goes on to say, "My father had all seven children work in his office at various times. He believed that we should understand how a family business worked from the ground up. We learned everything from filing, scheduling appointments, assisting patients, scheduling, and, as a medical student, assisting with surgeries. What I carried forward from my father's example was a confidence to meet with individuals in the business world and collaborate with them" (e-mail communication, January 2023).

Dr Gohara relied on colleagues for help. As she says, "I asked for help. In my experience, no one gets anywhere alone. I was not ashamed to ask for help with my, at the time, young children, or professional goals. Dermatology is comprised of a small group of people who are more like family members–family members who are willing to help!" (e-mail communication, January 2023).

I can say, unequivocally, that much of my success is due to having a very strong support network made up of my spouse, family, friends, and colleagues who supported, guided, and encouraged me along the way. There were times along my journey when I lost direction, wanted to give up, thought I was not worthy, did not see the light at the end of the tunnel, or imagined that I couldn't succeed.[10] Yet the people in my support network knew otherwise. I listened to them, heeded their advice, and leaned on them when necessary to restore my strength and renew my verve. Most successful women I speak with have these same thoughts of occasional self-doubt. I think that having these feelings is part of what makes us stronger, more driven in the end, and, perhaps, even more successful. When you realize that there are people who care about you and want to help you succeed, you don't want to let them down. And you don't want to let yourself down.

Always use the resources that you have at your disposal. Don't be afraid to ask for advice or words of wisdom from family, friends, colleagues, or mentors whom you trust. You might be surprised at how helpful they will be and how freely they share their resources and knowledge. Truly successful people tend to want to elevate others and help them succeed as well.

### Don't be afraid to do the hard work

Dr Piliang says, "The keys to success in the business of dermatology are similar to other fields: hard work, consistency, kindness and showing up. On repeat. Every day" (e-mail communication, February 2023).

According to Dr Day, "I have worked my way from the bottom up in many ways. I have worked in so many different jobs over the years that required so many different skill sets, and I did so much of my own administrative and daily work as I was growing my business. All of that has helped me understand what the business needs, what it means to be in every role I ask of my staff, and where I need to pay attention in order to streamline the work and optimize the patient experience. There's a climb up to the top for a reason. Every step builds muscle and learning, and those give strength and confidence to take the next step. Sometimes we slip, but that learning is important as well" (e-mail communication, January 2023).

Most of our patients, and even our staff, do not realize the inordinate number of hours we put in as successful businesswomen in dermatology. I am usually the last one to leave the office, but my work doesn't end then. I often spend hours at night and on the weekends not only working on charts but managing the office, signing the checks, reviewing the invoices and statements, planning the marketing strategy, researching treatments, perusing current literature, writing for publications, preparing for conferences, participating in society leadership zoom conferences, and so on. All of these responsibilities are hard in their own way, largely because they take time away from my family and social life. But they are responsibilities that I have chosen to undertake as the owner of a solo dermatology practice and as a physician leader. I feel that they have helped enlighten me and make me a better physician, business owner, boss, and colleague.

### Learn from your mistakes

Dr Day says, "In the beginning (I became successful) by failing a lot and by learning from my mistakes, as well as by listening to and learning from others smarter than me. As I grew it was more about seeing what worked, learning from that, tweaking it and doing more of the same" (e-mail communication, January 2023). Dr Carruthers agrees, saying, "I learned from my mistakes. I was never afraid to admit them and I asked for lots of advice" (text message communication, February 2023).

That theme prevailed in my interviews with successful businesswomen in dermatology. We all make mistakes along the way. Some are bigger and more costly in terms of time, money, or stress, but most of them are reversible, recoverable, or even rewarding when they lead you down another, better path.

I appreciate Dr Mariwalla's honesty when she says, "I made A LOT of mistakes. Running a successful business in dermatology isn't something that comes naturally but is something you evolve into. Having honest conversations with friends who are practice owners has helped. But mainly it has been keeping tabs on the journals so my knowledge base doesn't become outdated and then leaning into technology to help me run more efficiently. But basically, I only figured it out because I messed it up so many times. The key thing, however, is to make sure you are always a doctor first. When you lose sight of that, the whole thing goes down" (e-mail communication, February 2023).

### Make the most of each patient's experience

In the words of Dr Piliang, "Caring for your patients like they are your friends or family builds trust and loyalty. That reputation will have your phones ringing off the hook and your waiting rooms full" (e-mail communication, February 2023).

Allison Vidimos, MD, Chair of Cleveland Clinic's Department of Dermatology, Vice Chair of the Cleveland Clinic Dermatology and Plastic Surgery Institute, and member of the AAD Board of Directors, says "Success for our department of dermatology means supporting engaged and fulfilled staff, residents, fellows and support staff who truly enjoy their work and find reward in delivering skilled, cutting edge, empathetic care for our patients. Success encompasses educating our staff, trainees and medical students and performing innovative research to improve the quality and safety of our care. Success means highly satisfied patients" (e-mail communication, February 2023).

One of the best procedures I have incorporated into my practice is to make each patient feel welcome, special, and at-home from the moment they make first contact with our front office team until after they are home from their visit. My staff is friendly and trained according to the motto, "The answer is yes. Now what is the question." The office space is designed to feel comfortable and welcoming, clean, and professional to ensure patient confidence in the care we provide. After surgical procedures, I contact my patients to ensure their satisfaction. I also share with them my cell phone number so they can contact me if they need anything from me or my staff. Patients love the personal attention. I love knowing that, if my patients have a true concern, I can address it right away. Essentially, we try to imagine and walk through the patient experience from start to finish to ensure we are providing them with the best care we can.

## Success in Your Profession Outside of the Walls of Your Practice

### Decide what role you want to take in your specialty

Engaging in some way with your specialty can make it more meaningful to you, especially when you know you have a positive impact. There are many ways to get involved. For instance, if you like to teach but are in private practice, you can affiliate with a university and teach residents. Or you can apply to be a speaker at local, state, national, or international dermatology meetings. If you like advocacy, you can participate in the AAD Association's or American Society for Dermatologic Surgery Association's national advocacy efforts. If you like governance, you can apply to be on one of the national dermatology organizations' councils, committees, and task forces. Or you can join your local dermatology or medical associations and reach out to their leadership or administrators to find out how you can get involved. Local and state medical societies are always looking for interested physicians. You can also volunteer in your community, offering skin cancer screenings or lecturing on topics of interest to local residents.

### Find your niche

Dermatology is one of the few specialties that offers a diverse spectrum of subspecialties. Ideally and traditionally, you can decide what aspect of dermatology is most intriguing to you during residency and complete your training with a fellowship in your subspecialty of choice. If you love treating acne, make it a focus of your practice. If you really enjoy the challenge of treating pigmentary disorders, learn all you can about it and become an expert in the field. Learn and do what makes you happy, and your patients will follow.

According to Linda Stein Gold, MD, AAD Vice President and Division Head of Dermatology and Director of Dermatology Clinical Research at Henry Ford Hospital in Detroit, "I have become successful by abiding by the motto 'if there is a will, there is a way.' I have stepped out of my comfort zone to accept challenges and opportunities. Even if I felt unprepared, I overprepared so when the time came, I was the expert in the room" (e-mail communication, January 2023).

Personally, I have always enjoyed dermatologic surgery. When I consult with my patients, I always say, "My goal is to make it look like no skin cancer was ever there." In keeping with that aim, I developed and published, over the course of my career, innovative suturing techniques to avoid transepidermal sutures for more optimal surgical outcomes. My interest in suturing techniques filled a niche in our specialty, which led me to create the AAD's first hands-on suturing techniques course. Today, my focus is on beauty. Therefore, I studied the topic in depth and now lecture on it internationally.

Study or research it. Learn it. Teach it. Become the expert in it. Fill a niche. You can be the "go-to" person for whatever interests you most. Patients will come to you for your expertise. Dermatologists will benefit from your advice and knowledge. Giving back to our specialty by being a researcher and/or faculty member at educational meetings is hugely rewarding and a great way to become a leader in our specialty.

### Build relationships

Relationships you build with your colleagues and peers will also provide long-term value. They will be a valuable source of education, information-sharing, trouble shooting, understanding, and camaraderie. They might also serve as a good referral source. They will understand the struggles of dealing with difficult staff, challenging patients, and regulatory burdens. They will also relate to the pressures of balancing a happy home life with a busy work life.

Your family and friends are your most important relationships, and they deserve special attention. Unfortunately, however, these relationships are often the ones that suffer the most, perhaps because we assume they will always be there for us. The fact that, for most of us, family and friends are always there for us and can provide our greatest source of enjoyment is why these relationships should be fostered. No matter how busy you are, set aside even a few minutes a day or a few hours a week to connect in person, over the phone, or virtually with those you love. It will matter to both of you.

### What Does It Take to Be a Successful Businesswoman in Dermatology?

Success takes initiative, drive, determination, hard work, and the desire to succeed.

Deirdre Hooper summarized her journey to success well when she said, "I attribute the success I have to curiosity, hard work, and finding support networks that help me achieve goals. I am always open to new ideas. I read a LOT, I stay involved with professional societies, and I listen to trusted friends. I am super organized with my calendar and to-do list, and I give 100 percent effort to tasks I undertake. Finally, I delegate as much as I can!" (e-mail communication, February 2023).

### SUMMARY

Success is a personal construct that means something different to everyone. Successful businesswomen in dermatology know what type of practice they really want, and they create a plan to bring it to fruition. They align their business with their life and lifestyle, often choosing to live near their workplace. Most agree that it is important to surround themselves with people who support their goals and facilitate goal achievement. Although they often reluctantly accept support, they know when to delegate and how to delegate appropriately.

Successful businesswomen in dermatology are not afraid to do the hard work required to be successful and often feel that they gain knowledge and strength from the experience. When they make mistakes, they own up to them and learn from them. Most importantly, they agree that the patient is the focus of their practices, so they try to make the most of each patient's experience. They also agree that relationships with family, friends, and colleagues, as well as personal growth, are of utmost significance outside of their practices.

Being successful means looking inside yourself, figuring out who you are, what drives you, what you really want, and what you are willing to give up in order to get there. It takes soul-searching and perseverance. Be honest with yourself. Know what you are capable of achieving and go for it.

### DISCLOSURE
#### Financial Conflicts of Interest

None.

#### Professional Conflicts of Interest

Vice President-Elect, American Academy of Dermatology (AAD); Executive Committee, AAD; Board of Directors, American Society for Dermatologic Surgery; Board of Directors, Noah Worcester Dermatologic Society; Board of Directors, Florida Academy of Dermatology; Board of Directors, Florida Society for Dermatologic Surgeons; Chair, AMA Dermatology Section Council;

Past President, Florida Academy of Dermatology; Past VP, Women's Dermatologic Society.

## REFERENCES

1. Murrell DF, Ryan TJ, Bergfeld WF. Advancement of women in dermatology. Int J Dermatol 2011;50(5): 593–600.
2. Dyke LS, Murphy SA. How we define success: a qualitative study of what matters most to women and men. Sex Roles 2006;55:357–71.
3. Healthecareers. Available at: https://www.healthe careers.com/career-resources/career-opportunities/ dermatologys-many-fulfi. Accessed March 05, 2023.
4. Highland J. 7 Tips to start your private dermatology practice. Available at: https://miiskin.com/dermatology/ clinic-setup/starting-your-own-practice/. Accessed March 04, 2023.
5. Straus SE, Straus C, Tzanetos K. International campaign to revitalise academic medicine. Career choice in academic medicine: systematic review. J Gen Intern Med 2006;21(12):1222–9.
6. Castaldo A, Pittiglio R, Reganati F, et al. Access to bank financing and start-up resilience: a survival analysis across business sectors in a time of crisis. Manch Sch 2023;91(3):141–70.
7. Funding Circle. A physician's guide to medical practice loans. Available at: https://www.fun dingcircle.com/us/resources/medical-practice-finan cing/. Accessed 05 March, 2023.
8. Practice Management Center, American Academy of Dermatology Association. Available at: https:// www.aad.org/member/practice. Accessed March 04, 2023.
9. Collins LR, Jim C. Good to great: why some companies make the leap... and others Don't. New York: Harper Business; 2001.
10. Moskal E. Physicians experience impostor syndrome more often than other U.S. workers. Available at: https://med.stanford.edu/news/all-news/2022/09/ physicians-imposter-syndrome.html. Accessed March 05, 2023.

# Incorporating Cosmetic Procedures into Your Dermatology Practice

Lana L. Long, MD

## KEYWORDS

- Cosmetic procedures • Dermatology practice • $CO_2$ laser procedure • Platelet-rich plasma

## KEY POINTS

- Cosmetic procedures can be a nice addition to your dermatology practice. Do your homework, talk with your patients and have fun. Don't expect a huge profit increase as many devices and lasers are quite expensive with ongoing maintenance, service contracts and consumables.
- Set aside a certain block of time to see cosmetic patients and increase as you build up your practice. It's a diferent pace and you want to answer patients questions and not be rushed. Also there is no confusion of what is covered medically and what is cosmetic and self pay.
- Get proper training. Take a course at the AAD or ASDS, speak with a colleague doing cosmetic procedures and read articles and textbooks pertaining to the procedure you are thinking of adding to your practice.

Cosmetic procedures can be a nice addition to many different types of dermatology practices. It is part of our specialty, and I would encourage anyone interested to pursue adding a few procedures to their current practice.

Why perform cosmetic procedures? It can be esthetically pleasing for many dermatologists, there is a growing demand for esthetic procedures, and it is a source of additional increased revenue not tied to Medicare.

According to 2019 American Society for Dermatologic (ASDS) statistics, nearly 14 million treatments were performed by its members in 2019, including 3.5 million skin cancer treatments, 4 million injectables, 1 million body sculpting procedures, and 4 million laser and light treatments.[1]

It is nice to have an additional source of income not tied to Medicare rates. However, do not count on it be more financially rewarding than a fast-paced general dermatology practice. One great advantage of cosmetic procedures is the ability to raise fees to keep up with inflation, which is near impossible with insurance fixed to Medicare rates that do not keep up with inflation.

One major hurdle for a cosmetic practice is the upfront cost of the equipment. Additional warranties, maintenance, and consumables also need to be factored in. Make no mistake equipment manufacturers have tried to maximize their profit margins, often by necessitating expensive disposables.

On a different note, cosmetic patients can also be somewhat needy and have high and sometimes unrealistic expectations. You need to aware of, and avoid, patients with body dysmorphic disorder, who will never be happy with your efforts.[2]

Do not underestimate the value of your time. A general dermatologist's average income is $368,500 per year.[3]

If you perform patient care 40 hours per week and work 48 weeks a year, you generate a little under $200 per an hour. It takes at least 30 minutes to perform laser hair removal on a man's back or woman's legs. The value of your time, plus that of your equipment, and your staff's time (do not forget check in and check out) and additional profit must all be added to see if your prices for that procedure are realistic.

Private Practice, City Dermatology & Laser, 580 Walnut Street, Suite P-0160, Cincinnati, OH 45202, USA
E-mail address: Lanallong@yahoo.com

Dermatol Clin 41 (2023) 667–671
https://doi.org/10.1016/j.det.2023.05.005
0733-8635/23/© 2023 Elsevier Inc. All rights reserved.

Some procedures can be delegated, depending on the regulations of your state medical board. Check this early on if thinking about adding a new procedure. I recently hired someone with a more advanced degree to help with laser hair removal and non-ablative fractionated lasers, and it has freed up my time to do other procedures. I could not have done this with a medical assistant.

We truly are the experts in skin care, and dermatologists have pioneered many of the currently popular cosmetic procedures. We owe tremendous gratitude to Drs Jean and Alastair Carruthers for their innovation with cosmetic Botox use,[4] Dr Hal Brody and Dr Gary Monheit for their innovations with chemical peels,[5,6] and Dr Rox Anderson for the description of photothermolysis and current application to many of our laser procedures[7]

I currently practice 1 to 2 days of general dermatology and 2 to 3 days of cosmetic dermatology weekly. A busy general dermatology practice is an obvious fit for adding cosmetic procedures. Many of your existing medical patients likely ask about cosmetic procedures and would be interested if added to your practice. If you do a lot of surgery, a vascular laser and microneedling might be a good place to start to improve scars, though it can get difficult explaining why this service is an additional charge. Pediatric dermatologists might use a vascular laser for hemangiomas and warts and microneedling or chemical peels for acne scarring.

Some may choose to do primarily cosmetic dermatology. This might work if you are part of a larger group practice that refer patients to you. Most cosmetic dermatologists I know, also see some general dermatology, as this drives the cosmetic side of your practice. Talent is important, but it takes time to build up a busy cosmetic practice. You will be competing with many other individuals who have little or no formal training and patients may not be willing to pay for additional credentials. Most of my cosmetic patients are also medical patients or word of mouth referral from other patients, though I receive some from other doctors, including non-dermatologists.

*Setting aside a certain block of time* in the schedule for cosmetics is important. You want to do your best to stay on time and try not to overbook. The waiting room will be less crowded, and patients will be of a similar type. It is a slower pace and you do not want to act rushed. Perhaps start out with half of a day and build up as able. Fridays are my busiest cosmetic day. I see a lot of downtown professional patients who desire to have the weekend to recover from potential bruising or erythema.

*Look at your demographics*. I built my office downtown, where I was initially the only physician doing cosmetic procedures. My patients include a lot of attorneys, bankers, and federal worker as well as fortune 500 company employees such as P&G, Kroger, and GE. Cosmetic patients must have disposable income for their procedures. They value their time, and coming in for a fast, minimal downtime, in office procedure fits into their schedule. Early morning and lunch hours are particularly busy.

*Do some homework*. Ask your current patients which cosmetic procedures they are interested in. General dermatology patients frequently enquire about cosmetic procedures. I have a flyer with my procedures and prices and a video loop in the waiting room describing them. I also have a large notebook with a one-page description on my letter head of available procedures, before and after photos, and costs, in every examination room. I briefly discuss and send the information home with my patient if they ask about the procedure. Many general dermatology visits turn into cosmetic consultations! I will sometimes also send the information home with a medical patient when indicated. For example, rosacea or androgenetic alopecia patients to know the cosmetic options for their problems. I make it clear to patients that there are two sides of my practice and give information, but apply no pressure. Many of my patients are glad that I mentioned the cosmetic options and are pleasantly surprised by the costs. Others are not interested, and that's ok.

*Check out the competition*. Are there several cosmetic options in your area? What procedures do they offer? Are they well trained? Perhaps you and a colleague around the corner want to share a laser. A colleague in South Africa, Dr Pieter DuPlessis, shares a laser center with six other dermatologists. This way they all have the latest technology available but share the cost. What a great idea!

*Look at the start-up costs* when deciding which procedure to add. Not only the machine or material but also disposables and even on-going usage charges can make a procedure unprofitable. Newer device manufacturers have worked to extract maximum profit from their devices. Sometimes, devices based on older technology, for example, KTP lasers, work very well. These are solid state (more reliable) much less expensive and work well when used with polarized lenses, especially after an intense pulsed light or non-ablative laser treatment.

Neuromodulators and fillers are the home run of cosmetic procedures. They work consistently, give great results, and can be used on all skin types, and patients come back in on a regular schedule! The products can be purchased individually, and as such have a relatively low start-up cost. Chemical peeling, sclerotherapy, microneedling, and platelet-rich plasma (PRP) for androgenetic alopecia also all have relatively low start-up costs. The pharmaceutical representatives can be helpful in providing basic training and information.

*Do more homework*, lasers and devices are expensive, and many have consumables or usage cards that need to be purchased. It is like buying an expensive car, and you should test drive several! You want to look at three to four of the companies and have them bid the laser/device you are interested in. Look at the costs not only of the device and consumables but also maintenance agreements, ease of use, and time and staffing needed.

As mentioned above, the greatest cost in any cosmetic procedure is your time. Physicians tend to grossly underestimate the time it takes them to perform services. Make sure that the salesperson brings the device for you to try on a few patients or staff. Time yourself by the clock, including preparation time and postoperative instruction time. You will be surprised! Although you can expect to get faster with more experience, there is no way to speed up the laser recharge time.

Try to have the salesperson leave the device in your office for a few weeks to truly get a feel for it. First and foremost, you need to make sure it works; there is always a lot of hype around a new laser or device. You need to make sure that your patients can handle the discomfort and that you and your staff can readily use the device.

Before bringing a new procedure into my practice, I usually try it out on staff, family, and friends. I usually treat at no cost or for my supply costs. It helps you get comfortable with the procedure and also staff can discuss the new procedure first hand with your patients. You may not realize how many friends you have and I think this is one reason I have maintained such a great staff!

Some of the devices are quite large and occupy a lot of space, and some are more mobile and can be easily moved from room to room if necessary. A few still require a special electric supply, but most now plug into a regular electric receptacle. You also need to look at the payoff and return on investment. The laser companies will often give you a rough idea, but do not usually include overhead, maintenance agreements, disposables, or physician time in the equation, but always include your tax deductibility, which is never a good reason to buy something.

I also like to speak to my colleagues doing a lot of cosmetics to see which laser/device they purchased and how they like it. Never pay full price, there is frequently a show special or a demo unit available. If you have a trade in, this can also be helpful. I usually get 20% to 50% off the list price. You can also ask for a longer service contracts/warranties, which can be a significant expense (aim for 3 years), more training for you and staff, and extra cards or consumables. Many also have a marketing firm you can use to get the word out on your new purchase. They all have brochures to hand out to patients and waiting room banners. Leasing may be an option to look into as well.

*Proper training* is of utmost importance. You will get some basic training when you add a new procedure, but you want to be the best at what you offer. The American Academy of Dermatology (AAD) and the ASDS offer many hands-on courses. I have attended several, and highly recommend them.

Qualifications to perform some procedures is minimal and enforcement tenuous. I once met a medical assistant who worked for a plastic surgeon at a local course, who insisted that she was not a medical assistant, but instead an "injectologist." Dermatologists are highly trained and should charge more accordingly. I like to be at the higher end of the going rate. You do not want patients seeking a "Groupon" bargain; you want to be known as one of the best. There are many textbooks on cosmetic procedures which are helpful. Also, it is nice to spend a day or two with a colleague who does cosmetics, to see how the office is run, what procedures offered, and so forth.

*Be a dermatologist first*. I was referred a patient with an invasive melanoma that another non-dermatologist cosmetic laser office sent to me as it was not responding to laser treatments. On further inquiry, the doctor was an emergency Room (ER) physician who decided to open up a laser practice.

Women will often wear heavy makeup and hide large lentigos and other lesions. Biopsy anything that looks suspicious. Clear up the patient's acne before tackling acne scarring. Educate melasma patients about sunscreen and sun protection, because it may very well recur after expensive laser treatments!

Make sure that you are recommending the proper procedure. I saw a patient who underwent a $CO_2$ laser procedure by a plastic surgeon and was upset that she still had a lot of vascular lesions! Patients will often come in asking for what their friend had or what they read about in an article. Take time to analyze the patient to see if it a problem with skin tone, texture, lines, or volume. You know what you can help with and recommend appropriate treatment or refer to another specialist. When running through the options, I will sometimes recommend an eye lift, a face lift, tummy tuck, or something I do not do. I give the patient a sheet with a name and phone number of someone doing quality work in my area.

*Be prepared for cosmetic emergencies.* You must recognize and be prepared to treat cosmetic emergencies. These rare side effects need to be mentioned in your consent form. If using fillers, you need to have hyaluronidase on hand in case of a filler arterial occlusion. Avoiding danger zones or modifying technique in these areas is also important. Using injection cannulas used in certain areas may also decrease this risk.

If a patient receiving neuromodulators develops an eyelid ptosis, iopidine drops can be used for temporary relief until it normalizes. Patient selection and knowing where not to inject are most helpful in preventing this.

An overpowered laser can blister and settings must be immediately reduced. I frequently do a test area, particularly for darker skin types, with different settings in an inconspicuous area. The patient is instructed to call if any of the areas leave persistent redness, blisters, or hyperpigmentation. Any blistering should be treated with a potent topical steroid. Hyperpigmentation must be treated early and aggressively, with bleaching agents and ongoing sun protection.

Patients should also be given written pre- and post-care instructions. I include a topical postprocedure cream in the price of many procedures. This way, you know what they are using and more importantly that they are not using something on their skin which could cause irritation, allergy, infection, or impede healing.

I order topical and oral medications for the convenience of my patients and include this in the price of the procedure. Preoperatively I apply topical 2.5% lidocaine/2.5% prilocaine, which takes the sting out of many lasers and devices. I keep oral antibiotics and antivirals on hand to use for prophylaxis. Patients undergoing $CO_2$ laser procedures and microneedling are at high risk for reactivation of their herpes. The patient appreciates not having to stop at the drug store and is compliant.

*Always take photos before and after all procedures.* Patients are amazed that one eyebrow is slightly lower than the other before the neuromodulator! I try to gently point out any areas of asymmetry or small scars before a procedure. A review of the photos has changed an unhappy patient to a satisfied one on many occasions in my office.

I call the patient the day after any procedure, which takes some time to heal. It is nice to answer any questions, and the patient appreciates the individual attention. I have my contact number (personal cell phone) on my post-care sheets so the patient can easily call if they have a question or problem. We show patients' photos of what to expect during the healing phase and do our best to educate before the procedure.

*Patient comfort is important.* You do not need a fancy office, but a few thoughtful touches can go a long way. We provide make up removers and soft absorbent cloth towels for patients. We try to make the patients as comfortable as possible and have pillows and blankets available. If the procedure requires any gel, we place a nice beach towel on the examination table for the patient to sit on. We also have cloth gowns and cloth bathrobes for our patients. These items can be purchased relatively inexpensively online or at discount retail stores.

Certain patients are prone to faint, and I often inject neuromodulators with the patient lying down. Fillers require a larger needle and are thus more painful. I like to have patients in an examination chair which can be quickly placed in Trendelenburg position if the patient gets light headed. We have ammonia inhalant capsules in each room in case the patient has a vasovagal episode. Always tip into Trendelenburg first as restoring blood flow to the brain quickly remedies this. A bad vasovagal reaction with a seizure can ruin your day.

I always have a plan about how much neuromodulator and filler to inject in which location. I mark the injection sites and other anatomic landmarks with a white eye lining pencil. We sometimes use topical numbing agents or a nerve block if injecting into a sensitive area. We use small ice packs with our logo for 45 to 90 seconds before injecting filler. It is great marketing and we send the patient home with the ice pack to use at home.

*Pain control* is part of patient comfort, and you want to make the procedure as comfortable as possible for the patient. During injections, we offer patients a squeeze ball to take their mind off of what we are doing. Talkesthesia helps relax the patient, and I often enlist staff to chat with the patient so I can focus on the procedure.

Preoperatively I apply topical 2.5% lidocaine/ 2.5% prilocaine about 30 minutes before which takes the sting out of many lasers and devices.

We also offer nitrous oxide that the patient inhales it through a disposable tube. It is demand driven, so you do not need to worry about the quantity the patient inhales. It wears off in 10 minutes and patients can drive home or go back to work. It is not advisable to use in patients with asthma.

For IPL and laser hair removal, we use a chilling device with cold air to take the edge off. For non-ablative lasers and PRP, we offer topical anesthesia and use a chiller. Microneedling and microneedling with radiofrequency require topical numbing and we frequently add a chilling device. Ultherapy (high intensity focused ultrasound) and ablative lasers are more uncomfortable.

Forty-five minutes to an hour before a painful procedure I have the patients take 800 mg of ibuprofen in gel cap form, 2 gm of liquid acetaminophen, 10 mg of loratadine, and 60 mg of propranolol if there is no history of asthma. The gel cap and liquid forms are absorbed more quickly and help with pain control, the loratadine helps with swelling, and the propranolol helps with anxiety without sedation. At the same time, I apply topical 2% lidocaine and 2.5% prilocaine (EMLA) application for 30 to 45 minutes. The patients are free to drive themselves to the procedure and back home, as no sedation is used. I learned this very useful nonsedating method while visiting Dr Kevin Smith.[8]

We also use the air chiller and squeeze ball or vibration device.

*Marketing* is something new to a lot of us. Your current patients are the best to market to, as they are familiar with your office and hopefully like you and your staff. I have framed before and after pictures of the procedures offered in all of my examination rooms. I move them around 3 to 4 times yearly. Patients frequently inquire about the photos and we can do a quick consult with pricing.

Update your Web site to include the cosmetic procedures offered. Facebook and twitter are also good options to introduce your practice and procedures offered. You can ask patients to post reviews and have them sent to Google reviews or Yelp. You can sign up for Realself and post answers on the procedures offered. Patients often asked what's new, especially if they know you just returned from a conference. This is a perfect time to discuss your new laser, device, or procedure.

I have a one-page typed procedure sheet in a binder in all of my examination rooms. If I am doing a full skin check and they ask about fillers and cryolipolysis, then boom, give them a handout and quote.

A happy patient will refer their friends. Some businesses give out cards, where they get a free treatment or cash off after so many visits. I give a select group of patients 10% off and call them VIPs. This could be someone who comes frequently, your friends, or someone who works in your building. My business was slow after the holidays, so I have been sending a holiday card to existing patients, offering $50 off of their next cosmetic procedure, including another card of $50 off to give to a friend. It really helped fill in my schedule.

Of course, you can hire someone to do your marketing or get input of a marketing firm. This can be very costly, so do your homework. Get in writing what your goals are and how they can help you accomplish them.

Be creative, you can make your own short videos, have an open house to show your new procedures, and take your flyers around to other offices. The AAD offers a Practice Management book, Starting and Marketing a Dermatology Practice, which I have found helpful.

In summary, cosmetic procedures can be a nice addition to a general dermatology practice but do your homework and do not expect a huge increase in profits. Talk with your patients, see what they want, and have fun!

## CLINICS CARE POINTS

- There is a growing demand for cosmetic procedures. It can be an additional source or revenue not tied to Medicare, but don't expect a huge increase in profits.

## REFERENCES

1. American Society for Dermatologic Surgery. Available at: www.asds.net/Procedures -Survey. Accessed Jan 3 2023.
2. Phillips KA. Body dysmorphic disorder: the distress of imagined ugliness. Am J Psychiatry 1991;148(9): 1138–49.
3. Salary.com. Dermatologist Salary in the United States. Available at: https://www.salary.com/research/salary/alternate/dermatologist-salary. Accessed Jan 3 2023.
4. Carruthers A, Carruthers J. Botulinum Toxin Type A: History and Current Use in the Upper Face. Semin Cutan Med Surg 2001;20(2):71–84.
5. Monheit GD. The Jessner's and TCA Peel: a medium-depth chemical peel. J Dermatol Surg Oncol 1989; 15(9):945–50.
6. Brody H. Variations and Comparisons in Medium-Depth Chemical Peeling. J Dermatol Surg Oncol 1989;15(9):953–63.
7. Anderson RR, Parish JA. Selective Photothermolysis: precise microsurgery by selective absorption of pulsed radiation. Science 1983;220(4596):524–7.
8. Niamtu J, Smith KC, Carruthers J. Pain Control in Cosmetic Facial Surgery. Soft Tissue Augmentation 2008;127–41.

# From Geraniums to Guadalajara on the Virtues of Early Retirement

Jerry D. Smith, MD, FAAD[a,b,c],*

## KEYWORDS

• Retirement • Mexico • Volunteer physician • Saving for retirement

## KEY POINTS

- Start saving as much as you can as soon as you can.
- Start thinking about where you want to retire and visit those places on vacation.
- Think about hobbies or skills you'd like to develop in retirement.
- There is no need for expensive vacations while working. There will be plenty of time if you retire early.

Early on I decided I would retire as soon as I could, and after a 25-year practice, I retired at the age of 55 years. I am not alone in this decision.[1] Several factors led to that decision, and quite frankly, I have had no regrets. Not once have I woken up and said, "Damn I wish I could go to work today!"

## EARLY YEARS

Four months after Pearl Harbor (in 1942 for the historically illiterate), I was born in a village of 800 in Indiana. My dad was a tail gunner in a B24 Liberator until he was shot down in a bombing mission over Germany. He then spent 18 months in a German prisoner of war camp. My mom and I lived with her parents until he returned when I was about 4 years old.

As a child my maternal grandfather started growing geraniums from cuttings and selling them in his parents' general store. He was very successful at this and turned it into a business that put him through college. He went on to build the largest geranium greenhouse in the United States. A book was published about geraniums where he was cited as the "Geranium King."

I started working for him in his greenhouse for 25 cents an hour when I was in the 7th grade. I was a hard worker and often put in 70-h weeks. I started driving tractors at age 12 years, saved my money, and bought my first car when I was 14 years. I have learned a lot from working. Hard work has always paid off for me.

While in high school, I earned an Eagle Scout certificate (signed by Dwight Eisenhower!) was class valedictorian out of 27, and was a 4-year letterman in basketball. My intelligence and aptitude tests showed that I was qualified to be a really smart forest ranger!

### Wabash College

I was thinking about civil engineering and wanted to go to a technical school but my father decided I would go to Wabash College, a nearby private, academically rigorous, all male liberal arts school (Wabash is still all male and academically rigorous). He often bragged that my private education only cost him $500. I kicked in my need-based scholarship, jobs at the fraternity house where meals were included, laboratory assisting after

a University of Texas, Southwestern Medical Center, Dallas, TX, USA; b Medical Arts Clinic, Corsicana, TX, USA; c LCS Free Skin Cancer Screening Clinic, Ajijic, Jalisco, Mexico
* Corresponding author. Emiliano Zapata #113, Ajijic, Jalisco, 45920.
E-mail address: dosmotos@yahoo.com

Dermatol Clin 41 (2023) 673–678
https://doi.org/10.1016/j.det.2023.05.007
0733-8635/23/© 2023 Elsevier Inc. All rights reserved.

classes, summer jobs, and my working nights at the recreation center watching over rowdy high school students.

My college advisor, who was a power on campus, took me under his wing and guided me through the 4 years there. He gave me the job in his laboratory and lined up a full-ride graduate position at Vanderbilt University in biochemistry. Turns out he and the Geranium King were from the same little village!

As mentioned, I was a hard worker and made almost all A's. It was at the end of my junior year that it dawned on me I was going to spend the rest of my life in a laboratory and not the great outdoors with Smokey the Bear. Most of my classmates were premed, and because I had already taken those classes, one day I decided to go to Med School. I could live my own life working for myself and be out in nature anytime I wanted—not in a laboratory.

I called the Dean of the Indiana University Medical School to see if there was a way to get into the current year's class which started in less than a month. He listened to my story and said he'd get back to me in a couple of weeks. SURE, I thought. A few weeks later he contacted me and said there was a place for me. Small world, he also knew the Geranium King.

The Dean at Wabash was opposed to my leaving early and convinced me to stay for my senior year. I stayed and earned a Phi Beta Kapa membership and an honors diploma. In retrospect, I think I wasted a whole year.

## Indiana University Medical School

Having stupidly turned down the Medical School Dean's generous offer, I now had to apply on my own. There were over 3000 applicants for the 200 positions. My fraternity brother, the smartest guy I've ever known who may get a Nobel Prize in chemistry someday, was interviewed just before me.

As he came out of the interview, he was flushed, disturbed, and maybe even tearful? He said it was the worst experience of his life. I was worried!

The first question to me was, "What do you think you made on the Medical College Admissions Test (MCAT) test?" I did not really know, but the five interviewers were persistent, so I guessed the 90th percentile where I usually fell. They all LAUGHED. I had either flunked it or gotten 100%—both unlikely. The next question was, "What was it like growing up in a small town?" I answered that it was fun. I got to do a lot of things. For one, I had a pet raccoon. That excited them. I then had

question after question about that damned raccoon, until my half hour was up. I was subsequently accepted, and to this day, I can't explain it. They *did not* know the Geranium King.

Freshman year was the worst part of Med School. It was always too much to read, not enough sleep, learning the medical language with no free time (or at least not much), all the while working three jobs.

One of my jobs was to act as an intern one night a week at a private hospital. I was a first year medical student and really didn't know anything. This was in the days where you were unsupervised and "thrown into" the job. I recall intubating a patient with lung cancer whose tumor had eroded into the aorta. It was a bloody disaster. I was upset they did not have a "Do not Code," on this terminally ill patient and asked the nurse why, she just shrugged.

I also worked the "The Friday Night Knife and Gun Club" at the general hospital emergency room (ER). This is where I became a "real" doctor. I saw a lot of stuff I would rather forget.

My best job was as an ambulance attendant for a funeral home. It may sound like a conflict of interest, but because of their roomy interiors funeral hearses used to act as ambulances all over the United States.[2] I got to "attend" all the local racetracks and Indianapolis 500. I was able to get a lot of reading time sitting in that nice Cadillac limousine. I was in the pit "ambulance" at the 500 in 1966, when there was a 20 car crash on the first lap at the starting line. On the TV replay, TV you can see me, little guy in a white coat running from car to car checking on drivers—all were fine.[3] A little while later a driver came to the "ambulance' and said he was injured as he held up a bloody stump of a hand. It turned out that he already had an artificial hand and had just abraded where the prosthesis fit. It was still shocking.

It was during my junior year of medical school that I knew I was headed for a life I didn't like. Sleep deprivation, little free time, and some of the disgusting things I saw and did wore on me. I wanted out of poverty, but not this way. In the early 1970s, insurance companies were offering a starting salary of $160,000 a year for a lawyer with a medical degree. This was terrific pay with regular hours and without the gore. I decided that I would not do an internship, but instead would go straight into law school. Then, I did a 6-week rotation in dermatology.

Here was everything I want rolled up in one specialty. The professor was enthused and lined up a residency with John Knox at Baylor in Houston. I think they were friends. I had to do an internship, however. I was given a sheet of paper with 10 lines for my top 10 selections for a hospital. By that time, I had had my fill of Indiana weather, so I only filled out the top three choices—all in Hawaii.

### Internship: A Private Hospital in Honolulu

The first thing I did was buy a surfboard—every Indiana boy wanted to be a surfer back then. However, after I learned to surf I saw my first shark attack victim in person and found out that I didn't need to report it to the authorities because it would be bad for tourism. I sold my surfboard and bought a $100 stake in an old Star Class Olympic sailboat and learned to race. I crewed for a retired Army Colonel on his Star Class boat, and we had some success. He agreed to let me sail his boat, with him crewing for me, in the big Maritime Regatta at the Waikiki Yacht Club. I won my first regatta. The fire was lit.

### Residency Houston

On the first day of my residency, I was put in charge of the 15-bed Derm Ward at the Veterans Administration (VA) Hospital. Making rounds with my professor, Dr Ben Smith, I was dismayed see that 13 of my 15 beds housed leg ulcer patients, some of whom had been there had been there 2 or 3 years. "What am I supposed to do with all these leg ulcer patients?" I asked. Dr Ben said, "Why not try pinch grafts." "How do I do that?" "Look it up," he said. So off I went to the library. There I found only one reference. It was a small red pocket-sized book of less than 100 pages written by a surgeon right after the Civil War. The section on pinch grafts was one paragraph that basically said to pinch up some skin with one hand, shave it off with a razor blade and slide it off onto the wound. Period! It didn't sound difficult, so I decided to try it. Over the next 8 weeks, we grafted all the leg ulcers, and almost all healed in a month or so.

Dr Smith said I should publish my results, and overnight, I became, the world authority on pinch grafting leg ulcers.[4] Then, came invitations to speak and teach at dermatologic surgery (a new subspecialty at the time) workshops and other meetings. The dermatologic surgeons would all teach each other, so over the years I learned all their techniques and skills too. Dermatologic surgery was in its infancy, and I published many more papers.

I visited the Houston Yacht Club and found a racing fleet of Olympic Star Class boats and a skipper who was looking for a trained crew. There was another guy named Jerry Smith who raced yachts and got his name in the newspaper a lot.

My chairman, Dr Knox thought it was I, so I got a lecture about wasting time when I should be studying.

Following my residency, I went to Bethesda, Maryland, to fulfill my obligation to the Navy.

### US Navy

One day when I was an intern in Hawaii, the hospital administrator said the commanding officer at Pearl Harbor wanted me to come at 1 PM. I had been getting deferrals from going to Vietnam for about 5 years, and I could get an additional 3 years for residency if I enlisted.

Young physicians do not appreciate how traumatic and disruptive wars can be. (Editor's note; they also do not appreciate that health care workers, particularly doctors, can be drafted up age 45 years and perhaps older with no sexual discrimination into their 50s. They should also appreciate that dermatologists are high up on the list of desirable military physician specialties: https://medschoolinsiders.com/medical-student/doctor-draft/).

World War II was a highly patriotic endeavor because of the sneak attack on Pearl Harbor, but this wore off during the Korean War. The Vietnam War was decidedly unpopular. In addition, I knew of three of my medical school classmates who had already been killed in Vietnam.

The Admiral's office was the entire third floor of the administration building on Ford Island. I remember the windows all around and the beautiful navy-blue wall-to-wall carpet with a giant yellow US Navy insignia woven in the center where we stood facing each other. It was 1969, and the war was winding down, but we were still there, and I was going to get sworn in. It was just the two of us, and it went well until he said the part about going "anywhere and doing anything" that caused a problem.

*"Does that mean that I'm swearing that I will go to Vietnam?"*

*Yes.*

*"Then I can't do that because I'm not going to Vietnam."*

*"Then I can't swear you in."*

*That's okay; you called me.*

Silence—dead silence for I have no idea how long I stood there holding my left hand on the Bible and my right hand up in the air. Finally, he skipped that part and went ahead with the swearing in. Welcome to the US Navy. I still had 3 more years of exemption left for my dermatology residency and hoped the war would be over by then.

### In the Navy

I was one of six staff dermatologists at Bethesda National Navy Hospital. We each saw a light load of 10 to 15 patients a day. It was exciting having VIPs as patients. The most enjoyable ones were the fighter pilots—I had always wanted to be one.

One day a Supreme Court Justice came in with a bleeding tumor in the eyebrow, and I gave informed consent for the biopsy which could leave a scar. All went well, and I later saw the same Justice on the cover of a National News magazine with my scar on his eyebrow.

A middle-aged man came in 1 day with a White House referral. He had what some doctors (not I) call "Great Balls of Fire." It was a mess down there. I told him it was usually caused by stress (this was right in the middle of Watergate). He denied stress but took the medicine and left. Two days later his picture was on the front page of the Washington Post as a Watergate conspirator. No wonder!

Probably, the highlight of my time in Maryland was when Kenny Rogers came to a honkytonk in rural Maryland. The band had made it big in Houston and was going national and about to break up. We got there about 30 minutes early and the place was empty. I went to the bathroom in the rear of the building, and when I came out, there was a guy sitting alone in the dark. I said, "You from Houston?" knowing the band was. "Yep." "Well so am I." "Well sit down and have a beer with me," said Kenny Rogers. He was really down in the dumps and related all the problems of the band and personal misfortunes. People filled the joint and Kenny put on a great show.

I was elated when my 2-year active-duty commitment was complete and ready to finally begin my career.

### Medical Arts Clinic Corsicana, Texas 1974

I had selected Kerrville, Texas, outside San Antonio, as the place I wanted to practice, but Corsicana recruited me heavily. Our Corsicana regional Medical Center served the nine surrounding counties; we were only 1 hour south of Dallas. I had just learned Mohs in the Navy and the fresh-tissue technique from Ted Tromovitch in San Francisco. The dermatologist already in Corsicana there gave me half of his patients and all the surgery. I was busy from day 1.

We had no ER in the clinic, so we would get calls all day to see patients, and I did when I could. Then, we lost both ENTs, so I saw their patients

as well. It was a very busy year, and I was making a real living at last.

The clinic had hired an older RN to work for me, but she was not surgically trained, meaning I had to train her. When she retired after a year or 2, I told them that I wanted them to send me high school valedictorians, who were smart enough to go to college, but could not afford it. I trained them as medical assistants, and after a year, they were high functioning. They did most of the work. I was able to schedule patients every 5 minutes which was the approximate time I spent with each one. The "nurses" did all the rest. What they were able to do competently, I let them do. The patients averaged about 20 minutes total each in the office and waiting time was minimal.

We had certain standards which the patients seemed to enjoy.

1. We worked in or stayed late to see all patients who called in with an urgent problem.
2. All cancer follow-up visits were free unless new problems had arisen. They all got recalls at 12-, 6-, or 3-month intervals. Free visits seemed to keep them coming back, and I got all the new business when they had a problem.
3. I warranted what I did unless it was cancer. If I had to freeze a lesion, it was under warranty. This generated lots of good will and patient referrals.

Flying back to Dallas from an Academy of Dermatology Meeting, I sat with the department chairman of the Department of Dermatology, University of Texas Southwestern Medical School, Paul Bergstresser. I told him about my interest in teaching dermatologic surgery in residency programs. He agreed and we started the Dermatologic Surgery Clinic at Parkland Hospital in Dallas. We recruited other surgically inclined dermatologists to help staff it. It was an instant success, and I taught there until I retired.

On another flight from a Dermatologic Surgery workshop, I sat next to Ted Tromovitch, who had taught me fresh-tissue Mohs, and I told him I was closing most of my Mohs defects, which at the time was something of a secret and frowned on. He confessed that he had been doing the same and suggested that I publish on this topic which I did.[5]

### Retirement

After 25 years at my working very hard I retired at age 55 years. I could tell I was burning out. On my first day at work 25 years earlier I was taken to the business office and asked how much I wanted to withhold for my retirement plan. The max was $35,000 a year, so that's what I did. It had grown a lot. I thought I had saved enough money to last the rest of my lifetime, and I was ready for a change. This decision was not as casual as I make it seem. My kids were independent, and my house and all debts paid off. I have always been frugal and calculated how much I could spend if I lived to age 78 (now age 81!) assuming no more work and only small appreciation.

My wife Sharon and I spent the first few years motorcycle touring around the United States, then the world with another couple. We even wrote a book about it.

In the early 1970s I had read an article in the Dallas newspaper that said in the 1960s, 2500 hippies had moved to Ajijic, Mexico (1 hour south of Guadalajara) and were living under trees down by Lake Chapala.[6] The weather there may be the best in the world, hovering around 75° year-round. According to the morning news, all the hippies did was lie around all day drinking wine, playing guitars, singing, painting, weaving, and smoking weed. It occurred to me that if I would learn to weave, I would fit right in!

We toured all of Mexico before visiting Ajijic. We bought a house on the third day and soon made our Texas home our vacation home. We have been living there since 1998.

I was not completely sure I had saved enough money to last, so I wanted to keep my surgical skills sharp in case I had to go back to work.

I became a volunteer physician in Mexico. It is very difficult to get a medical license in Mexico, so I partnered with a Mexican physician and we ran a clinic that serviced the 20,000 American retirees on the shores of Lake Chapala. It was ironic that I had planned on volunteering to help poor Mexicans, but it wound up that 95% of my patients were old, rich gringos. I recruited two other dermatologists, and we charged the gringos the going rate (about one-third of Texas rates). We donated all the money to scholarship funds for Mexican college students. College is cheap for Mexicans in Mexico, and we were funded about 40 college students a year for over 15 years.

I had some memorable cases. One of my first patients was a middle-aged Caucasian man with a 6-month history of a quarter-sized ulcer on top of his head with a necrotic mass at the base. When we asked what the mass was, he said it was a sheep embryo that had been grafted there by a physician in Veracruz to heal the ulcer!

When I turned 70, I stopped surgery, and 3 years later, I quit working in the free clinic. I became a supervisor/consultant, and to this day, I continue to do house calls. Old time patients call my house to see if they can come over to show me something or another. I'm always happy to oblige.

### On Teaching

Over my years of training, I had many volunteer dermatologists who taught me many clinical pearls and made me a better doctor. For this reason, I have always thought compelled to do the same. I have been a Baylor Med School instructor, Georgetown Med School Associate professor while in the Navy, and University of Texas Southwestern professor (Parkland Hospital) in Dallas. I think teaching keeps you up to date and in retrospect, was one of the most gratifying things I have done.

One of my students who I taught dermatologic surgery was Dr Brett Coldiron, past president of the AAD and editor of this issue.

## HOBBIES

I learned at Wabash that I could do almost anything if I had the right book. I believe hobbies have made retirement rewarding. This is what I have learned in my life from hobbies.

- Fly fishing
- Antique clocks (over 40 restored)
- Cattle ranching (100 acres with 20 cows)
- Whitewater canoeing (vice president of the Dallas Downriver Club)
- Whitewater kayaking (236 miles down the Grand Canyon twice)
- Catamaran racing (won three national championships and was on the US sailing team the year I tried out for the Olympics)
- Golf after I retired. I finally shot par when I was 74 years. I was never very good.
- Karaoke. After dancing at a local karaoke country western place, I decided that I could sing better than half their singers so took up singing. It is thrilling to get a crowd fired up with a song.
- Flint knapping (growing up in Indiana), I have always loved arrowheads. At age 74 years, I found a book, and it took about 5 years of daily knapping to be able to make museum quality points.

In conclusion, I have now been retired longer than I worked in private practice. I have not run out of money and have a beautiful mountainside "villa" overlooking the largest natural lake in Mexico. Our house has no heating or AC since we don't need it. All in all, I am happy the way it all turned out. It has been a great trip from the geranium greenhouse to Guadalajara.

## DISCLOSURE

The author has nothing to disclose.

## REFERENCES

1. Wittenberg-Cox, A. Is The 'Great Resignation' Actually A Mass Retirement? Forbes. Available at: https://www.forbes.com/sites/avivahwittenbergcox/2021/11/16/the-great-resignationactually-a-mass-retirement/?sh=70562bc918ba. Accessed May 15 2023.
2. Gershon, L. When Ambulances Were Hearses. JSTOR Daily. Available at: https://daily.jstor.org/when-ambulances-were-hearses/. Accessed May 15 2023.
3. Graham Hill Crash Indy 500 1966. Indy 500 1966 Big Crash RARE ANGLE. Available at: https://www.google.com/search?q=you+tube+indy+500+1966+big+crash+angle&rlz=1C1AWFC_enMX876MX884&oq=you+tube+indy+500+1966+big+crash+angle&aqs=chrome..69i57j0i546l4.35644j0j7&sourceid=chrome&ie=UTF-8. Accessed May 15, 2023.
4. Smith JD, Holder WR, Smith EB. Pinch grafts for cutaneous ulcers. South Med J 1971;64(10):1166–71.
5. Smith JD. Surgical repair of defects resulting from the serial fresh-tissue technique of Mohs. J Dermatol Surg Oncol 1977;3(2):184–7.
6. Rogers, M. Ajijic: Mexico's expat paradise on the lake. USA Today. Available at: https://www.usatoday.com/story/travel/destinations/2018/01/22/ajijic-mexicos-expat-paradise-lake/1053332001/. Accessed May 15 2023.

# Why I'm Still Practicing

Richard G. Bennett, MD[a,b,*]

**KEYWORDS**

• Medicine • Part-time practice • Retirement

**KEY POINTS**

- Continuing to practice medicine beyond retirement age should be a personal choice.
- Everyone has some cognitive decline with aging, but the severity and progression vary individually.
- Although some specialty societies and hospital systems are suggesting cognitive testing after a certain age, such testing is not in wide use but may become more common.
- In the absence of objective evidence, forced retirement of physicians should be viewed as an infringement on their autonomy.

Practicing medicine is not easy. In fact, it is rather stressful. Patients expect you will never make a mistake, and the days I practice are filled with questions, problems, complaints, emotional collisions, requests, and the list goes on. It used to be that we were relatively well compensated for all this trouble. But lately, things have taken a turn for the worse. Insurance companies are undercompensating physicians, and our expenses continue to increase. The result is that to maintain a decent income, we are forced to work harder. Some people say, "work smarter, not harder," which makes me think maybe the smartest thing to do is not work at all.

There is an anecdotal story near the fin de siècle (1897) about the author and bon vivant Gertrude Stein. After graduating from Radcliff College, she enrolled at Johns Hopkins Medical School—an honor and accomplishment for a woman at that time. After spending over 3 years in medical school, she decided to resign. The dean pulled her into his office to inquire what prompted the resignation. He said she was incredibly gifted and would make an excellent physician. She had only one thing to say: "You really don't know what it is to be bored, do you?"

In contradistinction to Ms. Stein, I have never found practicing medicine boring. It is interesting to figure out a difficult diagnosis or to help a patient improve. There is always some battle to fight or differing medical opinions and advances to grapple with.

As a general equation, time plus energy equals accomplishment. Thus,

$$T + E = A$$

Your energy level declines with age and you must budget your time appropriately. Still, as you age you recognize what is really important, what needs to be done now, and gloriously what will go away on its own if ignored.

Following are some general thoughts regarding the "continue to work" versus the "retire early" dilemma.

## THE MISSION

For myself personally, medicine has always been about helping others. As long as I am healthy, this mission is my main priority. There is no reason to quit. Those who argue for early retirement are either bored (which seems hard to believe) or think the monetary rewards are not worth the time.

There are other goals I have regarding the mission. I train younger physicians who will go on and train others. My goal is to set a good

Conflicts of Interest: None.

[a] Division of Medicine (Dermatology), David Geffen School of Medicine, University of California, Los Angeles, Los Angeles, CA, USA; [b] Department of Dermatology, Keck School of Medicine, University of Southern California, Los Angeles, CA, USA

* Bennett Surgery Center, 1301 20th Street, Suite 570, Santa Monica, CA 90404.

*E-mail address:* drrgb@g.ucla.edu

example as a physician so that the new generation will emulate my behavior in the future.

Another goal with the mission is medical research and writing (such as this article). Engaging in medical research sharpens our minds as sharpening a sword. Conducted properly, it gives us a deeper understanding. Discussion of this research with my staff and fellows results in greater insight in medicine.

## AVOID BUREAUCRACY

To accomplish the mission, we cannot let others interpose themselves between ourselves and the patients. If one allows this to happen, it has a corrosive effect on medical practice and is a cause of work dissatisfaction. I have carefully cordoned myself off from bureaucracy as much as possible, struggling daily to prevent the fortress that is my office from being breached by administrators, bumbling middle managers, meddling bureaucrats, and physician colleagues who are more than willing to do their bidding. I realize not all physicians are able to do this. However, every physician should realize that rules made by lawyers, administrators, insurance companies, and the like are made to benefit themselves in some way and not the patients.

I remember once an incident where a resident had inadvertently injected fat into the orbit. Being at an outside clinic, the patient needed an emergency ophthalmic consultation. The problem was how to transport her to the hospital. We simply took her in my car rather than arranging some other medical transportation as the hospital required.

## PROVIDES CLOSE NETWORK OF LIKE-MINDED FRIENDS

Continuing to practice provides an ever-expanding network of friendships with other physicians who are still there for the daily battle. Such friendships with trusted colleagues are essential for providing an interesting and productive work environment.

The mindset of physicians in closed medical environments—such as HMOs or even university medical systems—is quite different than that of physicians in private practice. Physicians in closed medical systems develop a work shift mentality and exist to support a somewhat needless bureaucracy. Even worse, the bureaucracy promotes a monotone narrative regarding proper patient management. There is no doubt that physicians in these systems would want to retire early, often with a generous retirement fund.

## MANDATORY RETIREMENT

Physicians are privileged in that they are not under mandatory retirement rules, in contrast to some other professions. In fact, the Employment Act of 1967 prohibits mandatory retirement based on age. Nevertheless, Congress passed mandatory retirement ages for air traffic controllers (age 56 years), national park rangers (age 57 years), and commercial airline pilots (age 65 years). In addition, the FBI requires retirement at age 57 years.

Although physicians are allowed to work as long as they like, there are efforts, particularly in the surgical specialties, to assess physicians' functional competence.[1,2] This is based on the assumption that the aging physician many not recognize their own functional decline. If one works for a hospital or medical system, more scrutiny is likely and will undoubtedly increase in the future. Stanford medical center now requires cognitive testing every 2 years for physicians at the age of 75 years and older (which incidentally, may be discriminatory if not applied to all its physicians).[2]

William Osler, the preeminent physician at the turn of the century at Johns Hopkins, felt that physicians should retire at age 60 years.[3] He based this opinion on the fact that persons older than 60 years accomplished very little. In fact, he felt physicians older than 40 years accomplished very little.[4] This idea was subsequently disputed by others. Dorland (of Dorland's medical dictionary) refuted this idea by analyzing the records of 400 famous men between the ages of 40 and 60 years who produced significant accomplishments.[5] Brendan Gill, an editor for The New Yorker, chronicled the lives of famous people who made significant contributions well into their 80s such as Grandma Moses.[6]

## COGNITIVE DECLINE AND COMPETENCY

All of us who are older (I'm 78 years old as I write this) recognize that our memories are not as sharp as when we were younger. I now and then have to search for the appropriate word. This mild memory difficulty is part of the normal aging process.[7,8] Mild cognitive impairment is the term used to describe this change. Although progression from mild cognitive impairment to more severe cognitive problems is unpredictable, it is somewhat reassuring to know that brighter, better educated individuals may be at lower risk of severe cognitive decline.[9] Furthermore, many successful physicians have type A personalities and high "grit" scores.[1] Cognitive thinking is roughly divided into crystallized intelligence and fluid intelligence.[10] Crystallized intelligence is the result of acquired information and is preserved until old age.[11] Fluid intelligence, on the other hand, is the ability to solve new types of problems. Fluid intelligence begins to decline in middle age, which supports Osler's opinion that we rarely accomplish much after age 40 years.[3] Nevertheless, there is considerable variation in cognitive decline between individuals.

On recertifying examinations, older physicians do less well than younger physicians. Specifically older physicians do well on testing older knowledge (crystalized intelligence) but do less well on more recent knowledge.[12] This emphasizes the need to "stay up to date" in one's field because the growth medical knowledge is astounding and is estimated to 50% obsolete every 10 years.

As we age, questions about competency arise and even more questions are asked about how to test for competency. Older physicians argue that clinical experience gained by many years in practice helps in diagnosis and management.[11] If these physicians remain thorough and energetic, their experience will be beneficial. However, if older physicians rely on first clinical impressions alone, they could be more prone to take incomplete histories and acquire incomplete data that may lead to diagnostic errors.[13] Regardless, of the arguments regarding competency, there is a growing consensus that physicians and surgeons should be assessed for cognitive and functional skills as they get older.[1,2] Complicating this issue is that individuals age cognitively at different rates, and there are conflicting opinions on how to assess cognitive skills as well as physical and mental stamina, coordination, reaction time, and judgment that will result in appropriate care.

## OPERATIVE SKILLS

As I've gotten older, I've noticed a few things about surgeries that I perform. First, my operative time is increased; I'm not quite as fast as I once was. Although not dramatically different, things just take me longer and making decisions takes longer. Second, new techniques have replaced older techniques we used 25 to 30 years ago. Because I have helped to develop some of these new techniques keeping up with the progression of medical science has not been an issue for my practice. Most importantly my dermatologic surgery fellows have kept me abreast of the latest developments and are never afraid to correct or educate. It is important to let oneself be open to being corrected. This, of course, is one of the fellows' greatest joys, as it should be. Thus, I believe my skill set is fairly up to date. However, if I were in

solo practice, learning new techniques might be a problem because I would not have a younger colleague eager to point out any errors and try new techniques.

An interesting idea is testing physicians for situational awareness, similar to testing for airline pilots.[2] Such testing assesses not only knowledge but also reaction time in a real-world, 3-dimensional environment. Perhaps such testing is not too far away with the development of virtual reality.

## DELAY FULL RETIREMENT AND WORK PART TIME

Physicians often tend to work as long as they can, particularly in low-stress specialties. A physician is often attached to work, and his or her identity is often based on what they do and with whom they work. As such, it is difficult to flip the switch from full-time work to full-time retirement. Therefore, delaying or transitioning to full retirement has many advantages.

First, part-time work is convenient, as it provides some income so as not to deplete your personal or retirement savings. Second, it allows you to continue taking care of patients who have seen you for years and with whom you have developed friendships. Further, there is personal satisfaction as well as emotional stimulation through maintaining relationships with coworkers. Third, it keeps your mind sharp. Fourth, avoiding an excessive workload will avoid the intensity of long work hours and burnout, which can occur more quickly in older physicians.[1] Most physicians cut their workload between ages 60 and 70 years.[1]

Nevertheless, there probably is a time to retire because one cannot manage physically or mentally.

Part time work often does not work well for the "medical systems" mentioned previously. These systems are geared for full-time employed physicians. They view part-time physicians as a financial burden and unnecessary. Before a physician signs up to work for a "medical system," he or she should investigate their policy regarding part-time work and mandatory retirement.

## HOBBIES

To continue to work in medicine past retirement age, it is important to stay in shape and develop some hobbies. For me, I take piano lessons, swim, and read nonmedical books. The piano improves my dexterity and keeps my mind and fingers quick, which is necessary for the surgery I do. The swimming obviously keeps me in good cardiovascular condition and maintains my stamina. Reading, I find, helps with the research and medical writing that I do.

## WHAT I WOULD DO IF I FULLY RETIRED

I don't look at retirement as a negative life transition. One's purpose can evolve. I sometimes look with envy on my friends who are retired, especially who retired early. They have so much time to do other things than medicine. I imagine I would study and accomplish things outside of medicine. One always dreams about writing the definitive text in whatever, but the problem is it needs to come from our experience and if we are not actively practicing, the daily experience is not there and probably no longer the desire.

Of course, we can always travel, but I realized early the time to travel was when I was younger because one never knows whether one can physically accomplish this as we get older.

## ADVANTAGES OF FULLY RETIRING

There are several advantages to fully retiring. First, one has more time for oneself to do those things one has always wanted to do, such as read or travel. Secondly, there is less pressure. Remember practicing medicine is continuous pressure and requires energy. Being retired will lower your blood pressure and perhaps improve your cardiovascular disease if present. Third, retirement expands one's time. Remember our formula, time + energy = accomplishment. So we can still accomplish something even as one's energy wanes. Either way, maybe there needs to be a clearly defined endpoint. Maybe we should reserve retirement for when the thrill of working is gone and our energy falls to zero—unless there are medical disabilities complicating the situation.

Sadly, some physicians cannot retire and still maintain their lifestyle, either due to ignoring retirement planning or having legal monetary obligations.

## SUMMARY

As one of my patients said to me the other day, "you can't retire till I die." It is comments like these that keep me going. As long as I am physically able, I recommend staying in the game and continuing the mission. On second thought, I think I'll buy a lottery ticket on the way home tonight.

## CLINICS CARE POINTS

- As physicians age, cognitive decline occurs at a variable rate.
- Operative times may increase with older physicians.

## REFERENCES

1. Sataloff RT. Physicians and retirement. Ear Nose Throat J 2019;98(7):394–5.
2. Sataloff RT, Hawkshaw M, Kutinsky J, et al. The aging physician and surgeon. Ear Nose Throat J 2018; 95(4–5):1–17.
3. Hirshbein LD. William Osler and The Fixed Period: Conflicting Medical and Popular Ideas About Old Age. Arch Intern Med 2001;161(17):2074–8.
4. Viets HR. William Osler and" The Fixed Period". Bull Hist Med 1962;36(4):368–70.
5. Dorland W.A.N. What the World Might Have Missed: The Great Work Done by Men over Forty. *Century.* 1908.
6. Gill B. Late bloomers. New York: Artisan Books; 1998.
7. Adler RG, Constantinou C. Knowing—or not knowing—when to stop: cognitive decline in ageing doctors. Med J Aust 2008;189(11–12):622–4.
8. Petersen RC. Clinical practice. Mild cognitive impairment. N Engl J Med 2011;364(23):2227–34.
9. Rentz DM, Huh TJ, Faust RR, et al. Use of IQ-adjusted norms to predict progressive cognitive decline in highly intelligent older individuals. Neuropsychology 2004;18(1):38.
10. Cattell RB. Theory of fluid and crystallized intelligence: A critical experiment. J Educ Psychol 1963; 54:1–22.
11. Eva KW, Cunnington JP. The difficulty with experience: does practice increase susceptibility to premature closure? J Contin Educ Health Prof 2006; 26(3):192–8.
12. Caulford PG, Lamb SB, Kaigas TB, et al. Physician incompetence: specific problems and predictors. Acad Med 1994;69(10):S16–8.
13. Bieliauskas LA, Langenecker S, Graver C, et al. Cognitive changes and retirement among senior surgeons (CCRASS): results from the CCRASS Study. J Am Coll Surg 2008;207(1):69–78.

# UNITED STATES POSTAL SERVICE®
## Statement of Ownership, Management, and Circulation
### (All Periodicals Publications Except Requester Publications)

| 1. Publication Title | 2. Publication Number | 3. Filing Date |
|---|---|---|
| DERMATOLOGIC CLINICS | 000 – 705 | 9/18/2023 |

| 4. Issue Frequency | 5. Number of Issues Published Annually | 6. Annual Subscription Price |
|---|---|---|
| JAN, APR, JUL, OCT | 4 | $438.00 |

**7. Complete Mailing Address of Known Office of Publication** *(Not printer) (Street, city, county, state, and ZIP+4®)*

ELSEVIER INC.
230 Park Avenue, Suite 800
New York, NY 10169

Contact Person
Malathi Samayan
Telephone *(Include area code)*
91-44-4299-4507

**8. Complete Mailing Address of Headquarters or General Business Office of Publisher** *(Not printer)*

ELSEVIER INC.
230 Park Avenue, Suite 800
New York, NY 10169

**9. Full Names and Complete Mailing Addresses of Publisher, Editor, and Managing Editor** *(Do not leave blank)*

**Publisher** *(Name and complete mailing address)*

Dolores Meloni, ELSEVIER INC.
1600 JOHN F KENNEDY BLVD. SUITE 1600
PHILADELPHIA, PA 19103-2899

**Editor** *(Name and complete mailing address)*

Stacy Eastman, ELSEVIER INC.
1600 JOHN F KENNEDY BLVD. SUITE 1600
PHILADELPHIA, PA 19103-2899

**Managing Editor** *(Name and complete mailing address)*

PATRICK MANLEY, ELSEVIER INC.
1600 JOHN F KENNEDY BLVD. SUITE 1600
PHILADELPHIA, PA 19103-2899

10. Owner *(Do not leave blank. If the publication is owned by a corporation, give the name and address of the corporation immediately followed by the names and addresses of all stockholders owning or holding 1 percent or more of the total amount of stock. If not owned by a corporation, give the names and addresses of the individual owners. If owned by a partnership or other unincorporated firm, give its name and address as well as those of each individual owner. If the publication is published by a nonprofit organization, give its name and address.)*

| Full Name | Complete Mailing Address |
|---|---|
| WHOLLY OWNED SUBSIDIARY OF REED/ELSEVIER, US HOLDINGS | 1600 JOHN F KENNEDY BLVD. SUITE 1600 PHILADELPHIA, PA 19103-2899 |

11. Known Bondholders, Mortgagees, and Other Security Holders Owning or Holding 1 Percent or More of Total Amount of Bonds, Mortgages, or Other Securities. If none, check box ► ☐ None

| Full Name | Complete Mailing Address |
|---|---|
| N/A | |

12. Tax Status *(For completion by nonprofit organizations authorized to mail at nonprofit rates) (Check one)*
The purpose, function, and nonprofit status of this organization and the exempt status for federal income tax purposes:
☒ Has Not Changed During Preceding 12 Months
☐ Has Changed During Preceding 12 Months *(Publisher must submit explanation of change with this statement)*

PS Form **3526**, July 2014 *(Page 1 of 4 (see instructions page 4))* PSN: 7530-01-000-9931 PRIVACY NOTICE: See our privacy policy on www.usps.com.

---

| 13. Publication Title | | 14. Issue Date for Circulation Data Below |
|---|---|---|
| DERMATOLOGIC CLINICS | | JULY 2023 |

| 15. Extent and Nature of Circulation | | | Average No. Copies Each Issue During Preceding 12 Months | No. Copies of Single Issue Published Nearest to Filing Date |
|---|---|---|---|---|
| a. Total Number of Copies *(Net press run)* | | | 119 | 120 |
| b. Paid Circulation (By Mail and Outside the Mail) | (1) | Mailed Outside-County Paid Subscriptions Stated on PS Form 3541 (Include paid distribution above nominal rate, advertiser's proof copies, and exchange copies) | 85 | 82 |
| | (2) | Mailed In-County Paid Subscriptions Stated on PS Form 3541 (Include paid distribution above nominal rate, advertiser's proof copies, and exchange copies) | 0 | 0 |
| | (3) | Paid Distribution Outside the Mails Including Sales Through Dealers and Carriers, Street Vendors, Counter Sales, and Other Paid Distribution Outside USPS® | 21 | 28 |
| | (4) | Paid Distribution by Other Classes of Mail Through the USPS (e.g. First-Class Mail®) | 8 | 9 |
| c. Total Paid Distribution *(Sum of 15b (1), (2), (3), and (4))* ► | | | 114 | 119 |
| d. Free or Nominal Rate Distribution (By Mail and Outside the Mail) | (1) | Free or Nominal Rate Outside-County Copies included on PS Form 3541 | 4 | 0 |
| | (2) | Free or Nominal Rate In-County Copies included on PS Form 3541 | 0 | 0 |
| | (3) | Free or Nominal Rate Copies Mailed at Other Classes Through the USPS (e.g. First-Class Mail) | 0 | 0 |
| | (4) | Free or Nominal Rate Distribution Outside the Mail (Carriers or other means) | 1 | 1 |
| e. Total Free or Nominal Rate Distribution *(Sum of 15d (1), (2), (3) and (4))* ► | | | 5 | 1 |
| f. Total Distribution *(Sum of 15c and 15e)* ► | | | 119 | 120 |
| g. Copies not Distributed *(See Instructions to Publishers #4 (page #3))* ► | | | 0 | 0 |
| h. Total *(Sum of 15f and g)* ► | | | 119 | 120 |
| i. Percent Paid *(15c divided by 15f times 100)* ► | | | 95.81% | 99.17% |

* If you are claiming electronic copies, go to line 16 on page 3. If you are not claiming electronic copies, skip to line 17 on page 3.

PS Form **3526**, July 2014 *(Page 2 of 4)*

| 16. Electronic Copy Circulation | Average No. Copies Each Issue During Preceding 12 Months | No. Copies of Single Issue Published Nearest to Filing Date |
|---|---|---|
| a. Paid Electronic Copies ► | | |
| b. Total Paid Print Copies (Line 15c) + Paid Electronic Copies (Line 16a) ► | | |
| c. Total Print Distribution (Line 15f) + Paid Electronic Copies (Line 16a) ► | | |
| d. Percent Paid (Both Print & Electronic Copies) (16b divided by 16c × 100) ► | | |

☒ I certify that 50% of all my distributed copies (electronic and print) are paid above a nominal price.

17. Publication of Statement of Ownership

☒ If the publication is a general publication, publication of this statement is required. Will be printed ☐ Publication not required.
in the OCTOBER 2023 issue of this publication.

| 18. Signature and Title of Editor, Publisher, Business Manager, or Owner | | Date |
|---|---|---|
| *Malathi Samayan* | | 9/18/2023 |

Malathi Samayan - Distribution Controller

I certify that all information furnished on this form is true and complete. I understand that anyone who furnishes false or misleading information on this form or who omits material or information requested on the form may be subject to criminal sanctions (including fines and imprisonment) and/or civil sanctions (including civil penalties).

PS Form **3526**, July 2014 *(Page 3 of 4)* PRIVACY NOTICE: See our privacy policy on www.usps.com.

# Moving?

## Make sure your subscription moves with you!

To notify us of your new address, find your **Clinics Account Number** (located on your mailing label above your name), and contact customer service at:

**Email: journalscustomerservice-usa@elsevier.com**

**800-654-2452** (subscribers in the U.S. & Canada)
**314-447-8871** (subscribers outside of the U.S. & Canada)

**Fax number: 314-447-8029**

**Elsevier Health Sciences Division**
**Subscription Customer Service**
**3251 Riverport Lane**
**Maryland Heights, MO 63043**

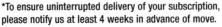

ELSEVIER

Printed and bound by CPI Group (UK) Ltd, Croydon, CR0 4YY

08/05/2025

01864749-0015